TYPE 1
DIABETES COOKBOOK
FOR KIDS

(A HEALTHY AND FRIENDLY DIET FOR KIDS WITH TYPE 1 DIABETES)

FLORY ADAMS

Contents

INTRODUCTION

Hey! We found the recipes

Jane, a 7-year-old girl, was the pride of Mandy's family. She and Jane both had a passion for cooking, and they frequently spent their weekends experimenting in the kitchen and preparing delectable meals for the family. But after learning that Jane had Type 1 diabetes, Mandy's entire world was thrown upside down. Mandy first worried about the impact this would have on her daughter's life and their cooking endeavors. She was devoted to helping Jane manage her condition while yet enabling her to eat the foods she cherished. Mandy started looking for recipes that were tasty and healthy, and she started making minor changes to their favorite foods. To discover the ideal combination of flavor and nutrition, she substituted high-sugar items for low-sugar equivalents and tried new ones.

Mandy and Jane were able to establish a schedule that worked for them despite some early difficulties. Together, they continued to prepare meals, and Jane learned how to meticulously monitor her blood sugar levels. Jane was able to eat her favorite dishes without worrying about blood sugar increases when they tried new recipes they loved. Mandy and Jane became further closer as time passed. Their love of cooking and experimentation only grew as they became one other's support system. Mandy was pleased with their progress and their ability to manage this new phase of their life together. In the end, Mandy understood that the most crucial thing was to never give up and to consistently look for a solution. She and Jane were still able to cook and make memories in the kitchen despite Jane's diabetes because of their love and support for one another.

In addition to teaching children a variety of skills, cooking with kids is a wonderful method to teach them about food and its origins. A great way to teach your diabetic child about how different foods can affect their blood sugar levels and to get them started on carb counting is to get them involved in meal preparation. Furthermore, it is a wonderfully enjoyable way to spend an afternoon with your child.

Cookbook for kids with Type 1 diabetes is one that is made especially for children. It includes diabetic children-friendly, nutritious, and balanced recipes. This cookbook's recipes are made to help kids manage their diabetes while still ensuring they eat wholesome meals and indulge in their favorite foods. This cookbook may also offer advice and recommendations on controlling diabetes, choosing healthy meals, and portion control.

CHILDREN WITH TYPE 1 DIABETES

The immune system of the body targets and kills the cells that make insulin, a hormone that controls blood sugar levels, in type 1 diabetes, a chronic illness. In order to restore the lost insulin and control their blood sugar levels, persons with type 1 diabetes must require insulin injections or an insulin pump. Children with type 1 diabetes require regular blood sugar monitoring and insulin dose modifications based on food intake, physical activity, and other factors. Children with type 1 diabetes can enjoy healthy, active lives with the right care.

SYMPTOMS

Type 1 diabetes in children typically manifests quickly and may cause the following symptoms:

- heightened thirst
- frequent urine and possible bedwetting in a kids who has completed toilet training
- severe hunger
- loss of weight
- Fatigue
- Intolerability or altered behavior
- A fruity breath smell

NUTRITION FOR CHILDREN WITH TYPE 1 DIABETES

1. CHOOSE THE RIGHT CARBOHYDRATES

In our diet, carbohydrates are a crucial source of energy. Starchy carbs and sugars are the two main categories of carbohydrates.

- Starchy carbohydrates content includes cereals, bread, potatoes, pasta, rice, and noodles.
- Sugar include: Table sugar (sucrose), lactose (the sugar included in dairy products), and fructose are examples of sugars (the sugar found in fruit)

The two main categories of starchy carbohydrate are:

- Unrefined wholegrain carbohydrates, which include whole meal bread and brown rice.
- Refined carbohydrates, which include white bread, white rice, and goods manufactured with white flour.

Rapid energy release from refined carbs can raise blood glucose levels. Wholegrain, unprocessed carbs release their energy gradually, and this maintains stable blood sugar levels. A diet rich in slow-release carbs, which are important providers of energy and nutrients, is recommended for children with diabetes. Additionally, some carbohydrates work better than others at extending the feeling of fullness after eating.

2. CHOOSE THE RIGHT KIND OF FAT:

Nutritionist categorize the "good fat" as:

- Healthy Monosaturated Fats
  These are primarily found in avocados, almonds, canola oil, olive oil, and canola.

- Polyunsaturated Fat
  Vegetable oils and margarines like sunflower, safflower, corn, and soybean oil include omega-6 fats. Fish high in oil, such as salmon, fresh tuna, sardines, and mackerel, are the main sources of omega-3 fats. Linseed (flaxseed) and its oil, canola oil, and soybeans are examples of plant sources.

Nutrionist categorize the "bad fat" as:

- Saturated Fat
  This can be found in full-fat dairy products (such as cheese, yogurt, milk, and cream), lard, ghee, and fatty meats, including pastry, cakes, cookies, coconut oil, and palm oil, as well as sausages and burgers.

- Trans Fat

These are made through the process of hydrogenation, which is used by food manufacturers to turn vegetable oils into semi-solid fats. They are also found in small amounts naturally in meat and dairy products.

Trans fats behave like saturated fat in the body even if they are technically unsaturated based on chemical analysis. Indeed, according to some studies, they are even worse for you than saturated fat.

3. REPLACE SALT WITH GOOD FLAVORING

CINNAMON

- Try adding cinnamon to stir-fries and other meat recipes, casseroles and stews. It might also aid in controlling blood sugar.

MUSTARD

- Mash potatoes with whole-grain mustard, or flavor cheese sauce with a dash of mustard powder.

HORSERADISH

- Grated Horseradish can be used as a sandwich spread when combined with mayonnaise.

GINGER

- Use as a salad dressing, salsa, or stir-fry sauce. It pairs well with flavors from meat, fish, or shellfish.

PEPPERCORNS

- It comes in a variety of colors; try pink, green, and Sichuan peppercorns in addition to black ones.

4. FIBER

fiber is crucial for kids with type 1 diabetes:

- Controlling blood sugar levels and lowering the risk of hyperglycemia is made possible by fiber's ability to slow down the digestion and absorption of carbohydrates.
- Weight control: Fiber, which is low in calories and can make you feel full, can assist with weight control and lower the risk of obesity, a common consequence of type 1 diabetes.
- Bowel regularity: Children with type 1 diabetes who may encounter changes in their digestion owing to drugs or high blood sugar levels may develop constipation, which is a frequent issue. Fiber can help control bowel movements and avoid constipation.

5. SUGAR INTAKE

NOT NO SUGAR, BUT LOW SUGAR

Two prevalent misconceptions are that eating too much sugar leads to diabetes and that persons with diabetes should stay away from every kind of sugar. In actuality, the impact of sugar on your blood glucose level depends on how much, in what form, and with which other meals you eat it.

Large portions of foods that are a concentrated source of natural sugar, such as fruit juice and dried fruit, should be avoided by people with diabetes. Small amounts of sugar are acceptable, especially when they are paired with high-fiber foods (which helps to slow down how quickly it is taken into the bloodstream). Although desserts, cookies, cakes, and candy are not strictly prohibited

A low-calorie or calorie-free sweetener might be the best choice, however, if you only need to sweeten a food without adding bulk. Information about the various choices is provided below:

TABLE SUGAR

Controlling your intake is crucial because 1 spoonful of sugar has 46 calories. Be mindful that switching another sweetener may not always work because sugar has other qualities besides sweetness that can influence a recipe's success.

HONEY

Compared to table sugar, using honey has minimal health benefits. Since honey is denser and so has a few more calories per spoonful, you often use less of it because it is also slightly sweeter.

FRUTOSE

Although it browns more quickly than table sugar, you can use it in the same ways. You may just need to lower the cooking temperature by 75°F (25°C). Its advantages include having a lower GI than table sugar and requiring less of it to get the same sweetness.

SACCHARIN

Since this sugar substitute has no calories, it can be used in foods that are cooked at high temperatures. It cannot be used in place of sugar in baking though because it is 300 times sweeter and does not share the same characteristics.

SUCRALOSE

This calorie-free sweetener, which is made from sugar but is not recognized as sugar by the body, has no impact on blood glucose levels. It is 600 times sweeter than sugar and incredibly heat resistant.

6. VEGETABLES

Incorporating vegetables into the diet of children with type 1 diabetes is important for several reasons:

1. Nutritional benefits: Vegetables are a good source of vitamins, minerals, and fiber that are essential for overall health and development. They also provide carbohydrates, which are the primary energy source for the body.

2. Blood sugar control: Vegetables have a low glycemic index, meaning they do not cause rapid spikes in blood sugar levels. This can help children with type 1 diabetes manage their glucose levels more effectively.

3. Variety in diet: Including a variety of vegetables in the diet can provide

different nutrients and flavors, making meals more enjoyable and helping to prevent boredom.

4. Disease management: Eating a diet rich in vegetables has been shown to reduce the risk of chronic diseases, including heart disease and some types of cancer. This can be especially important for children with type 1 diabetes, who have an increased risk of these conditions.

In conclusion, incorporating vegetables into the diet of children with type 1 diabetes is important for their overall health and well-being.

RECIPES

BREAKFAST RECIPES

Healthy Egg Muffins with Lean Turkey Bacon Recipe:

Preparation Time: 20 minutes

Cooking Time: 20 minutes

Servings: 6

Ingredients:

- 6 large eggs
- 6 slices of lean turkey bacon
- 1/2 cup diced bell peppers
- 1/2 cup diced onion
- 1/2 cup diced mushrooms
- Salt and pepper, to taste

Instructions:

1. Preheat the oven to 375°F (190°C). Grease a muffin tin with cooking spray.
2. Cook the turkey bacon in a pan until crispy, then chop into small pieces.
3. In a separate pan, sauté the bell peppers, onions, and mushrooms until soft.
4. In a large mixing bowl, whisk together the eggs and add the bacon, pepper mixture, salt and pepper. Mix well.
5. Pour the egg mixture into the muffin tin, filling each cup about 2/3 of the way.
6. Bake for 20-25 minutes, or until the eggs are set and the tops are lightly golden.
7. Serve hot and enjoy!

Nutritional Information (per serving):

Calories: 150

Protein: 12g

Fat: 11g

Carbs: 4g

Fiber: 1g

Benefit of the diet:

This healthy egg muffin recipe is a great option for those following a low-carb or high-protein diet. The eggs are a rich source of protein and healthy fats, while the veggies add fiber and essential vitamins and minerals. The lean turkey bacon provides a source of protein while being lower in fat than regular bacon. This recipe is an easy, nutritious and convenient option for a quick breakfast or snack.

Egg sandwich

Preparation Time: 5 minutes

Cooking Time: 5 minutes

Servings: 1

Ingredients:

- 2 large eggs
- 2 slices of whole grain bread
- 1 slice of cheese (optional)
- Salt and pepper, to taste
- Cooking spray

Instructions:

1. Crack the eggs into a bowl and beat well with a fork.
2. Heat a non-stick pan over medium heat and spray with cooking spray.
3. Pour the beaten eggs into the pan and scramble until fully cooked.
4. Toast the whole grain bread in a toaster.
5. Assemble the sandwich by placing the scrambled eggs on one slice of toast, adding the cheese slice (if using), and topping with the other slice of toast.
6. Serve hot and enjoy!

Nutritional Information (per serving):

Calories: 300

Protein: 19g

Fat: 15g

Carbs: 24g

Fiber: 5g

Benefit of the diet: This egg sandwich recipe is a simple, nutritious and satisfying breakfast option for children with diabetes. The whole grain bread provides fiber, complex carbohydrates, and essential vitamins and minerals, while the eggs are a rich source of protein and healthy fats. The cheese (optional) adds flavor and creaminess. The balanced combination of protein, fiber, and healthy fats helps to regulate blood sugar levels, making this an ideal breakfast choice for those with diabetes.

Sweet Potato and Chicken Sausage Hash Recipe:

Preparation Time: 10 minutes

Cooking Time: 20 minutes

Servings: 4

Ingredients:

- 1 large sweet potato, peeled and diced
- 1 cup diced onion
- 1 cup diced bell pepper
- 4 oz. chicken sausage, sliced
- Salt and pepper, to taste
- Cooking spray

Instructions:

1. Heat a large skillet over medium heat and spray with cooking spray.

2. Add the sweet potato and cook until tender, about 10 minutes.

3. Add the onion, bell pepper, and chicken sausage to the skillet and continue to cook until the vegetables are soft and the sausage is browned, about 10 minutes.

4. Season with salt and pepper to taste.

5. Serve hot and enjoy!

Nutritional Information (per serving): Calories: 180 Protein: 12g Fat: 7g Carbs: 20g Fiber: 3g

Benefit of the diet: This sweet potato and chicken sausage hash recipe is a delicious and nutritious option for people with diabetes. Sweet potatoes are a low-glycemic index food, meaning they help regulate blood sugar levels, while chicken sausage provides lean protein. The combination of protein, fiber, and healthy carbohydrates in this dish makes it an ideal breakfast or brunch choice for those with diabetes. Additionally, the added bell peppers and onion provide essential vitamins and minerals, making this dish a well-rounded and nutritious option.

Vegetable Omelet Recipe:

Preparation Time: 10 minutes

Cooking Time: 10 minutes

Servings: 1

Ingredients:

- 3 large eggs
- 1/4 cup diced bell pepper
- 1/4 cup diced onion
- 1/4 cup diced tomato
- Salt and pepper, to taste
- Cooking spray

Instructions:

1. Crack the eggs into a bowl and beat well with a fork.

2. Heat a non-stick pan over medium heat and spray with cooking spray.

3. Add the bell pepper, onion, and tomato to the pan and cook until tender, about 5 minutes.

4. Pour the beaten eggs into the pan and scramble until the eggs are set, about 5 minutes.

5. Season with salt and pepper to taste.

6. Serve hot and enjoy!

Nutritional Information (per serving):

Calories: 200

Protein: 16g

Fat: 12g

Carbs: 8g

Fiber: 2g

Benefit of the diet: This vegetable omelet is a nutritious and delicious option for people with diabetes. The eggs provide protein and healthy fats, while the bell pepper, onion, and tomato add fiber, vitamins, and minerals. This omelet is low in carbohydrates, making it a great breakfast or brunch option for those with diabetes. The combination of protein, fiber, and healthy fats helps to regulate blood sugar levels and keep you feeling full and satisfied throughout the morning. Additionally, this omelet is a quick and easy option that can be customized with your favorite vegetables, making it a versatile and convenient choice for those with busy schedules.

Zucchini & Parmesan Baked Omelet Recipe:

Preparation Time: 10 minutes

Cooking Time: 25 minutes

Servings: 2

Ingredients:

- 4 large eggs
- 1 medium zucchini, grated
- 1/4 cup grated Parmesan cheese
- 1/4 tablespoon salt
- 1/4 tablespoon black pepper
- 1 tablespoon olive oil
- Cooking spray

Instructions:

1. Preheat the oven to 375°F (190°C).
2. Grate the zucchini and set aside.
3. In a large bowl, beat the eggs and add the grated zucchini, Parmesan cheese, salt, and pepper. Mix well.
4. Heat the olive oil in a 9-inch (23 cm) oven-safe pan over medium heat and spray with cooking spray.
5. Pour the egg mixture into the pan and cook for 2-3 minutes, until the bottom is set.
6. Transfer the pan to the oven and bake for 20-25 minutes, or until the top is golden brown and the eggs are fully set.
7. Serve hot and enjoy!

Nutritional Information (per serving):

Calories: 250

Protein: 14g

Fat: 20g

Carbs: 4g

Fiber: 1g

Benefit of the diet: This zucchini and Parmesan baked omelet is a tasty and nutritious option for people with diabetes. The eggs provide protein and healthy fats, while the zucchini adds fiber and essential vitamins and minerals. The Parmesan cheese adds flavor and texture, while the olive oil provides heart-healthy monounsaturated fats. This omelet is low in carbohydrates, making it a great breakfast or brunch option for those with diabetes. The combination of protein, fiber, and healthy fats helps to regulate blood sugar levels and keep you feeling full and satisfied throughout the morning. Additionally, this omelet is easy to prepare and can be customized with your favorite vegetables, making it a versatile and convenient choice for those with busy schedules.

Sweet Potato Toast Recipe:

Preparation Time: 5 minutes

Cooking Time: 10 minutes

Servings: 1

Ingredients:

- 1 medium sweet potato
- Salt and pepper, to taste
- 1 tablespoon almond butter
- 1 tablespoon chopped nuts (optional)
- Fresh fruit (optional)

Instructions:

1. Preheat the oven to 400°F (200°C).

2. Wash the sweet potato and slice it lengthwise into 1/4-inch (0.5 cm) thick slices.

3. Place the sweet potato slices on a baking sheet and season with salt and pepper to taste.

4. Bake in the oven for 10-12 minutes, or until the slices are tender and lightly browned.

5. Spread almond butter over the sweet potato slices and top with chopped nuts and fresh fruit, if desired.

6. Serve hot and enjoy!

Nutritional Information (per serving):

Calories: 200

Protein: 5g

Fat: 12g

Carbs: 2

Fiber: 4g

Benefit of the diet:

This sweet potato toast is a tasty and nutritious option for people with diabetes. The sweet potato provides fiber, vitamins, and minerals, while the almond butter provides healthy fats and a source of protein. The nuts and fruit add texture and flavor, while also providing essential nutrients. This toast is a good source of carbohydrates, making it a great breakfast or brunch option for those with diabetes. The fiber in the sweet potato helps regulate blood sugar levels and keeps you feeling full and satisfied throughout the morning.

Oatmeal Breakfast Cookies Recipe:

Preparation Time: 10 minutes

Cooking Time: 15 minutes

Servings: 12

Ingredients:

- 1 cup quick-cooking oats
- 1/2 cup almond flour
- 1 tablespoon baking powder
- 1/4 tablespoon salt
- 1/2 cup unsweetened applesauce
- 1/2 cup almond butter
- 1/2 cup brown sugar
- 1 large egg
- 1 tablespoon vanilla extract
- 1/2 cup raisins
- 1/2 cup chopped nuts (optional)

Instructions:

1. Preheat the oven to 350°F (180°C). Line a baking sheet with parchment paper.

2. In a medium bowl, mix together the oats, almond flour, baking powder, and salt.

3. In a large bowl, beat together the applesauce, almond butter, brown sugar, egg, and vanilla extract until smooth.

4. Add the dry ingredients to the wet ingredients and mix until just combined.

5. Fold in the raisins and chopped nuts, if desired.

6. Using a cookie scoop, drop spoonful of dough onto the prepared baking sheet.

7. Bake for 12-15 minutes, or until the edges are lightly browned and the center is set.

8. Allow the cookies to cool on the baking sheet for 5 minutes before transferring to a wire rack to cool completely.

9. Serve and enjoy!

Nutritional Information (per serving):

Calories: 220

Protein: 6g

Fat: 15g

Carbs: 20g

Fiber: 3g

Benefit of the diet: These oatmeal breakfast cookies are a tasty and nutritious option for people with diabetes. The oats provide fiber, while the almond flour and almond butter provide healthy fats and a source of protein. The brown sugar and raisins add sweetness, while the chopped nuts add texture and flavor. These cookies are a moderate source of carbohydrates, making them a great breakfast or snack option for those with diabetes. The fiber in the oats helps regulate blood sugar levels and keep you feeling full and satisfied throughout the morning. Additionally, these cookies are a quick and easy option that can be made in advance and stored for later, making them a convenient choice for those with busy schedules.

Healthy Morning Glory Gingerbread Recipe:

Preparation Time: 10 minutes

Cooking Time: 30 minutes

Servings: 9

Ingredients:

- 1 cup whole wheat flour
- 1 tablespoon baking powder
- 1 tablespoon cinnamon
- 1 tablespoon ground ginger
- 1/4 tablespoon ground nutmeg
- 1/4 tablespoon ground allspice
- 1/2 cup unsweetened applesauce
- 1/2 cup molasses
- 1/2 cup brown sugar
- 1 large egg
- 1 tablespoon vanilla extract
- 1/2 cup grated carrots
- 1/2 cup raisins
- 1/2 cup chopped walnuts (optional)

Instructions:

1. Preheat the oven to 350°F (180°C). Grease an 8x8-inch (20x20 cm) baking pan.
2. In a medium bowl, mix together the flour, baking powder, cinnamon, ginger, nutmeg, and allspice.
3. In a large bowl, beat together the applesauce, molasses, brown sugar, egg, and vanilla extract until smooth.
4. Add the dry ingredients to the wet ingredients and mix until just combined.
5. Fold in the grated carrots, raisins, and chopped walnuts, if desired.
6. Pour the batter into the prepared baking pan.
7. Bake for 25-30 minutes, or until a toothpick inserted into the center of the bread comes out clean.
8. Allow the bread to cool in the pan for 10 minutes before transferring to a wire rack to cool completely.
9. Serve and enjoy!

Nutritional Information (per serving):

Calories: 220

Protein: 5g

Fat: 5g

Carbs: 40g

Fiber: 3g

Benefit of the diet: This Healthy Morning Glory Gingerbread is a tasty and nutritious option for people with diabetes. The whole wheat flour provides fiber and vitamins, while the applesauce and molasses provide natural sweetness. The brown sugar and raisins add a touch of extra sweetness, while the grated carrots and chopped walnuts add texture and flavor. This gingerbread is a moderate source of carbohydrates, making it a great breakfast or snack option for those with diabetes. The fiber in the whole wheat flour and grated carrots helps regulate blood sugar levels and keep you feeling full and satisfied throughout the morning. Additionally, this gingerbread is a quick and easy option that can be made in advance and stored for later, making it a convenient choice for those with busy schedules.

Children Breakfast Casserole Recipe:

Preparation Time: 10 minutes

Cooking Time: 20 minutes

Servings: 4

Ingredients:

- 4 large eggs
- 1/4 cup milk
- 1/4 tablespoon salt
- 1/4 tablespoon black pepper
- 1/4 cup shredded cheddar cheese
- 1/4 cup chopped vegetables (such as bell peppers, onions, mushrooms)
- 4 thin slices of lean ham or turkey bacon, chopped
- Non-stick cooking spray

Instructions:

1. Preheat oven to 375°F (190°C).
2. In a large bowl, whisk together the eggs, milk, salt, and pepper.
3. Stir in the cheese, vegetables, and chopped ham or turkey bacon.
4. Coat four children oven-safe ramekins with non-stick cooking spray.
5. Pour the egg mixture evenly into each of the ramekins.
6. Bake for 15-20 minutes, or until the egg is set and the top is lightly golden brown.
7. Serve hot and enjoy!

Nutritional Information (per serving):

Calories: 170

Protein: 12g

Fat: 12g

Carbs: 3g

Fiber: 1g

Benefit of the diet: These Children Breakfast Casseroles are a great option for people with diabetes. The eggs provide high-quality protein and healthy fats, while the vegetables add fiber and nutrients. The use of lean ham or turkey bacon adds flavor and protein, while the shredded cheese adds richness. This breakfast casserole is low in carbohydrates, making it a great option for those with diabetes. The combination of protein and fiber helps regulate blood sugar levels and keep you feeling full and satisfied throughout the morning.

Yogurt and Blueberry Parfait Recipe:

Preparation Time: 5 minutes

Servings: 1

Ingredients:

- 1 cup plain Greek yogurt
- 1/4 cup blueberries
- 1/4 cup granola
- 1 tablespoon honey (optional)

Instructions:

1. In a tall glass or parfait cup, layer 1/3 of the Greek yogurt on the bottom.
2. Sprinkle 1/3 of the blueberries over the yogurt.
3. Sprinkle 1/3 of the granola over the blueberries.
4. Repeat the layering process two more times, ending with a layer of granola.
5. Drizzle with honey, if desired.
6. Serve immediately and enjoy!

Nutritional Information (per serving):

Calories: 250

Protein: 20g

Fat: 9g

Carbs: 25g

Fiber: 2g

Benefit of the diet: This Yogurt and Blueberry Parfait is a great option for people with diabetes. Greek yogurt is a low-carb, high-protein source of dairy that can help regulate blood sugar levels and keep you feeling full and satisfied. Blueberries are a low-carb fruit that is high in antioxidants and other essential nutrients. The granola adds a crunchy texture and some carbohydrates, but is balanced by the fiber in the blueberries and the protein in the yogurt. This parfait is also a quick and easy breakfast option that you can enjoy on-the-go. Additionally, the optional drizzle of honey can add a touch of natural sweetness for those who prefer it.

Low Carb Apple Cider Donut Holes Recipe:

Preparation Time: 20 minutes

Cook Time: 10-12 minutes

Servings: 12

Ingredients:

- 1 cup almond flour
- 1/4 cup coconut flour
- 1 tablespoon baking powder
- 1 tablespoon ground cinnamon
- 1/4 tablespoon nutmeg
- 1/4 tablespoon salt
- 3 large eggs
- 1/4 cup unsweetened applesauce
- 1/4 cup unsweetened almond milk
- 1/4 cup apple cider

- 1 tablespoon vanilla extract
- 1/4 cup erythritol or other low-carb sweetener
- Optional: 1 tablespoon cinnamon-sugar substitute for topping

Instructions:

1. Preheat the oven to 350°F and line a muffin tin with paper liners.
2. In a medium-sized bowl, whisk together the almond flour, coconut flour, baking powder, cinnamon, nutmeg, and salt.
3. In a separate bowl, beat the eggs and then stir in the applesauce, almond milk, apple cider, vanilla extract, and erythritol.
4. Gradually mix the dry ingredients into the wet mixture until well combined.
5. Using a cookie scoop or spoon, fill each muffin cup about 2/3 full with the batter.
6. Bake for 10-12 minutes, or until a toothpick inserted into the center of a donut hole comes out clean.
7. Allow the donut holes to cool for 5 minutes in the muffin tin, then transfer them to a wire rack to cool completely.
8. Optional: sprinkle the cinnamon-sugar substitute on top of the donut holes.
9. Serve and enjoy!

Nutritional Information (per serving, 1 donut hole):

Calories: 70

Protein: 3g

Fat: 6g

Carbs: 4g

Fiber: 2g

Benefit of the diet: These Low Carb Apple Cider Donut Holes are a tasty and healthy breakfast or snack option for people with diabetes. Almond flour and coconut flour are both low-carb flours that are high in fiber, protein, and healthy fats. The addition of apple cider and cinnamon gives the donut holes a delicious apple flavor without adding too many carbohydrates. Using a low-carb sweetener, such as erythritol, helps to keep the overall carb count low. This recipe is also a gluten-free option for those with gluten sensitivities. Enjoy these donut holes as a sweet treat without having to worry about spikes in blood sugar levels.

Low Carb Waffles Recipe

Preparation Time: 10 minutes

Cook Time: 5-7 minutes per waffle

Servings: 4 (2 waffles per serving)

Ingredients:

- 1 1/2 cups almond flour
- 1/4 cup coconut flour

- 2 tablespoon erythritol or other low-carb sweetener
- 2 tablespoon baking powder
- 1/2 tablespoon cinnamon
- 1/4 tablespoon salt
- 4 large eggs
- 1/2 cup unsweetened almond milk
- 1/4 cup melted unsalted butter or coconut oil
- 1 tablespoon vanilla extract

Instructions:

1. Preheat a waffle iron.
2. In a medium-sized bowl, whisk together the almond flour, coconut flour, erythritol, baking powder, cinnamon, and salt.
3. In a separate bowl, beat the eggs and then stir in the almond milk, melted butter or coconut oil, and vanilla extract.
4. Gradually mix the dry ingredients into the wet mixture until well combined.
5. Spoon the batter into the preheated waffle iron, filling it to just below the rim.
6. Cook the waffles for 5-7 minutes, or until they are golden brown and crispy.
7. Repeat with the remaining batter, keeping the finished waffles warm in a 200°F oven.

8. Serve with your favorite low-carb toppings, such as fresh berries, whipped cream, or sugar-free syrup.

Nutritional Information (per serving, 2 waffles):

Calories: 400

Protein: 15g

Fat: 36g

Carbs: 12g

Fiber: 8g

Benefit of the diet: These Low Carb Waffles are a delicious and healthy breakfast option for people with diabetes. Almond flour and coconut flour are both low-carb flours that are high in fiber, protein, and healthy fats. The use of a low-carb sweetener, such as erythritol, helps to keep the overall carb count low, while still providing a touch of sweetness. The addition of eggs and almond milk provides protein and healthy fats, making these waffles a satisfying and filling meal. This recipe is also a gluten-free option for those with gluten sensitivities.

Zero Carb French Toast Recipe:

Preparation Time: 10 minutes

Ingredients:

- 2 large eggs
- 1/4 cup heavy cream
- 1 tablespoon vanilla extract
- 1/2 tablespoon cinnamon

- 1/4 tablespoon salt
- Butter or oil for frying
- 2 slices of zero carb bread (e.g. almond flour bread)

Instructions:

1. In a shallow dish, whisk together eggs, heavy cream, vanilla extract, cinnamon, and salt.
2. Heat a frying pan over medium heat and add butter or oil.
3. Dip the bread slices in the egg mixture, ensuring that both sides are well coated.
4. Fry the bread slices in the pan until golden brown on both sides, about 2-3 minutes per side.
5. Serve hot with your choice of toppings.

Nutritional Information (per serving):

- Calories: 243
- Total Fat: 22g
- Saturated Fat: 11g
- Total Carbohydrates: 3g
- Fiber: 2g
- Protein: 9g

The benefit of following a zero carb diet is that it can lead to weight loss and improved insulin sensitivity, as it eliminates all sources of carbohydrates and sugar. However, it is important to note that a zero carb diet may be challenging to follow in the long-term and may lack essential nutrients. It is always best to consult a healthcare professional before starting any new diet.

Frittata Recipe for Diabetic Diet

Preparation Time: 10 minutes

Cooking Time: 20 minutes

Servings: 6

Ingredients:

- 8 large eggs
- 1/2 cup milk
- Salt and pepper to taste
- 1 tablespoon olive oil
- 1 onion, chopped
- 2 cloves garlic, minced
- 1 cup cherry tomatoes, halved
- 1 cup baby spinach leaves
- 1/2 cup grated cheddar cheese
- Fresh parsley for garnish (optional)

Instructions:

1. In a large bowl, beat together the eggs, milk, salt, and pepper.
2. In a large non-stick skillet, heat the olive oil over medium heat. Add the chopped onion and minced garlic, and cook until softened, about 5 minutes.
3. Add the halved cherry tomatoes and baby spinach leaves to the skillet.

Cook until the spinach has wilted and the tomatoes have softened, about 2 minutes.

4. Pour the beaten egg mixture into the skillet, spreading the vegetables evenly. Cook for 5 minutes without stirring.

5. Sprinkle the grated cheddar cheese over the frittata.

6. Transfer the skillet to a preheated oven and bake for 10 minutes, or until the cheese is melted and the frittata is set.

7. Remove the frittata from the oven and let it cool for a few minutes.

8. Serve the frittata hot, garnished with fresh parsley, if desired.

Nutritional Information (per serving, with 1 slice of frittata):

- Calories: 200
- Fat: 15g
- Protein: 12g
- Total Carbohydrates: 5g
- Fiber: 2g
- Net Carbs: 3g

Benefits of a Low-Carb Diet: This frittata is a great option for children with diabetes, as it is relatively low in carbohydrates and high in protein. The eggs used in this recipe provide a source of high-quality protein, which can help to regulate blood sugar levels. Additionally, the olive oil used in this recipe is a good source of healthy fats,

which can help to improve overall health and prevent the development of related health problems. The vegetables used in this frittata (onion, garlic, cherry tomatoes, and baby spinach) are high in fiber and provide a source of slow-digesting carbohydrates, which can help regulate blood sugar levels. The cheese used in this recipe is a good source of calcium, which is important for overall health and wellbeing.

Zucchini Pancake Recipe for Diabetic Diet

Preparation Time: 10 minutes

Cooking Time: 15 minutes

Servings: 4

Ingredients:

- 2 medium zucchinis, grated
- 2 large eggs
- 1/4 cup almond flour
- Salt and pepper to taste
- 1/4 teaspoon garlic powder
- 1/4 teaspoon onion powder
- 1 tablespoon olive oil
- Fresh parsley for garnish (optional)

Instructions:

1. In a large bowl, mix together the grated zucchinis, eggs, almond flour, salt, pepper, garlic powder, and onion powder.

2. In a large non-stick skillet, heat the olive oil over medium heat.

3. Spoon about 1/4 cup of the zucchini mixture into the skillet for each pancake.

4. Cook the pancakes for 2-3 minutes on each side, or until golden brown.

5. Repeat the process with the remaining zucchini mixture, adding more olive oil to the skillet as needed.

6. Serve the zucchini pancakes hot, garnished with fresh parsley, if desired.

Nutritional Information (per serving, with 2 pancakes):

- Calories: 150
- Fat: 12g
- Protein: 7g
- Total Carbohydrates: 6g
- Fiber: 2g
- Net Carbs: 4g

Benefits of a Low-Carb Diet: These zucchini pancakes are a great option for children with diabetes, as they are relatively low in carbohydrates and high in healthy fats and protein. The almond flour used in this recipe is a good source of healthy fats, which can help to improve overall health and prevent the development of related health problems. The eggs used in this recipe provide a source of high-quality protein, which can help to regulate blood sugar levels. The zucchinis used in this recipe are a good source of fiber, which can help regulate blood sugar levels. Additionally, zucchinis are a low-carb vegetable, making them an ideal ingredient for children with diabetes. The use of herbs and spices, such as garlic and onion powder, in this recipe can add flavor without adding additional carbohydrates.

HEALTHY AND DELICIOUS LUNCH BOX SNACK RECIPE

Type 1 Banana Oat Muffin Recipe:

Preparation Time: 20 minutes

Serving: 2 persons

Ingredients:

- 1 cup rolled oats
- 1 cup all-purpose flour
- 1 tablespoon baking powder
- 1/2 tablespoon baking soda
- 1/4 tablespoon salt
- 1/4 tablespoon cinnamon
- 1 large egg
- 1/4 cup unsalted butter, melted
- 1/4 cup brown sugar
- 1 ripe banana, mashed
- 1/2 cup almond milk

Instructions:

1. Preheat your oven to 375°F (190°C).

2. Line a muffin tin with paper liners.

3. In a large mixing bowl, combine the oats, flour, baking powder, baking soda, salt, and cinnamon.

4. In a separate bowl, whisk together the egg, melted butter, brown sugar, mashed banana, and almond milk.

5. Add the wet ingredients to the dry ingredients and stir until just combined.

6. Divide the batter evenly between the muffin cups, filling each about 2/3 full.

7. Bake for 18-20 minutes or until a toothpick inserted into the center of a muffin comes out clean.

8. Let the muffins cool for 5 minutes before removing from the tin and serving.

Nutritional Information (per serving):

- Calories: 128
- Total Fat: 7g
- Saturated Fat: 4g
- Total Carbohydrates: 16g
- Fiber: 2g
- Protein: 3g

The benefit of incorporating oats into your diet is that they are a rich source of soluble fiber, which can help regulate blood sugar levels and lower cholesterol. Additionally, using almond milk instead of dairy milk can help reduce overall calorie and fat intake. However, it is important to keep in mind that even healthy muffins can still contain added sugars and should be consumed in moderation as part of a balanced diet.

Zero Carb Granola Bars Recipe:

Preparation Time: 10 minutes

Cooking Time: 20 minutes

Total Time: 30 minutes

Ingredients:

- 1 cup almond flour
- 1/2 cup coconut flour
- 1/2 cup unsweetened coconut flakes
- 1/4 cup flaxseed meal
- 1/4 cup chia seeds
- 1/4 cup sunflower seeds
- 1/4 cup pumpkin seeds
- 1/2 tablespoon salt
- 1/2 tablespoon cinnamon
- 1/2 cup melted coconut oil
- 1/2 cup almond butter
- 1 tablespoon vanilla extract

Instructions:

1. Preheat oven to 350°F (175°C). Line an 8x8 inch baking pan with parchment paper.

2. In a large mixing bowl, combine almond flour, coconut flour, coconut flakes, flaxseed meal, chia seeds, sunflower seeds, pumpkin seeds, salt, and cinnamon.

3. In a separate mixing bowl, whisk together melted coconut oil, almond butter, and vanilla extract.

4. Add the wet ingredients to the dry ingredients and mix until well combined.

5. Transfer the mixture to the prepared pan and press firmly to form an even layer.

6. Bake for 20 minutes, or until the edges are golden brown.

7. Remove from oven and allow to cool completely in the pan.

8. Cut into bars and serve.

Nutritional Information (per bar):
Calories: 178 Fat: 17g Carbohydrates: 4g Protein: 5g

Benefits of a Zero Carb Diet:

- Helps to promote weight loss

- Reduces inflammation

- Increases energy levels

- Improves mental clarity

- Supports heart health by reducing the risk of cardiovascular diseases.

Low Carb Slice and Bake Crackers Recipe:

Preparation Time: 10 minutes

Cooking Time: 20 minutes

Total Time: 30 minutes

Ingredients:

- 1 cup almond flour
- 1/4 cup flaxseed meal
- 1/4 cup sesame seeds
- 1/2 tablespoon baking powder
- 1/2 tablespoon salt
- 1/4 cup melted butter
- 2 eggs

Instructions:

1. Preheat oven to 350°F (175°C). Line a baking sheet with parchment paper.

2. In a large mixing bowl, combine almond flour, flaxseed meal, sesame seeds, baking powder, and salt.

3. Add melted butter and eggs to the dry ingredients and mix until well combined.

4. Divide the mixture in half and shape each half into a log. Wrap each log in plastic wrap and freeze for at least 30 minutes.

5. Remove from freezer and slice each log into 1/4 inch rounds.

6. Place the rounds on the prepared baking sheet and bake for 15-20 minutes, or until golden brown.

7. Remove from oven and allow to cool completely on the baking sheet.

Nutritional Information (per cracker): Calories: 68 Fat: 6g Carbohydrates: 2g Protein: 3g

Benefits of a Low Carb Diet:

- Helps to promote weight loss
- Reduces the risk of heart disease
- Improves blood sugar control
- Increases satiety
- Supports healthy liver function.

Banana and Whole Grain Toast Recipe:

Preparation Time: 5 minutes

Cooking Time: 5 minutes

Total Time: 10 minutes

Ingredients:

- 2 slices of whole grain bread
- 1 ripe banana
- 1 tablespoon cinnamon
- 1 tablespoon honey (optional)
- 1 tablespoon butter or margarine

Instructions:

1. Toast the whole grain bread to desired level of crispiness.

2. Meanwhile, in a small bowl, mash the ripe banana with a fork.

3. Mix in the cinnamon and honey (if using).

4. Spread the mashed banana mixture onto each slice of toast.

5. Top with a small amount of butter or margarine.

6. Serve immediately and enjoy!

Nutritional Information (per serving):

Calories: 227

Fat: 5g

Carbohydrates: 44g

Protein: 8g

Benefits of a Whole Grain Diet:

- Supports heart health

- Helps to regulate digestion

- Maintains stable blood sugar levels

- Supports healthy weight management

- Promotes a healthy immune system.

Salmon Cakes with Dill Aioli Recipe:

Preparation Time: 20 minutes

Cooking Time: 10 minutes

Total Time: 30 minutes

Serving: 2 persons

Ingredients: For the salmon cakes:

- 1 can (14 oz) boneless, skinless salmon, drained and flaked

- 1/4 cup breadcrumbs

- 1 egg

- 1 green onion, finely chopped

- 1 tablespoon lemon juice

- 1 tablespoon Dijon mustard

- 1 tablespoon dried dill

- 1/2 tablespoon salt

- 1/4 tablespoon black pepper

- 1 tablespoon olive oil

For the dill aioli:

- 1/2 cup mayonnaise

- 2 cloves garlic, minced

- 1 tablespoon lemon juice

- 1 tablespoon dried dill

- Salt and pepper, to taste

Instructions:

1. To make the salmon cakes: In a large mixing bowl, combine the flaked salmon, breadcrumbs, egg, green onion, lemon juice, Dijon mustard, dried dill, salt, and pepper. Mix until well combined.

2. Using your hands, form the mixture into 4-6 cakes.

3. Heat the olive oil in a large skillet over medium heat. Add the salmon cakes and cook until golden brown

on both sides, about 4-5 minutes per side.

4. To make the dill aioli: In a small bowl, whisk together mayonnaise, garlic, lemon juice, dried dill, salt, and pepper until well combined.

5. Serve the salmon cakes with the dill aioli on the side.

Nutritional Information (per salmon cake with 1 tablespoon of aioli): Calories: 223 Fat: 17g Carbohydrates: 4g Protein: 15g

Benefits of a Salmon-Based Diet:

- Supports heart health
- Promotes brain health
- Increases energy levels
- Supports joint health
- Helps to regulate digestion

Classic low carb donut recipe

Preparation Time: 10 minutes

Cooking Time: 5 minutes

Total Time: 15 minutes

Ingredients:

- 1 cup almond flour
- 1/4 cup coconut flour
- 1/4 cup sweetener (such as erythritol or stevia)
- 1 tablespoon baking powder
- 1/4 tablespoon salt
- 2 eggs
- 1/4 cup unsweetened almond milk
- 1 tablespoon vanilla extract
- Oil for frying (such as coconut or avocado oil)

Instructions

1. In a large mixing bowl, whisk together the almond flour, coconut flour, sweetener, baking powder, and salt.

2. Add in the eggs, almond milk, and vanilla extract and mix until well combined.

3. Heat a small amount of oil in a large saucepan over medium heat.

4. Using a cookie scoop or spoon, drop the batter into the hot oil in 2-tablespoon portions.

5. Fry the donuts until golden brown, about 2-3 minutes per side.

6. Remove from the oil and drain on a paper towel-lined plate.

7. Serve immediately, or allow to cool and store in an airtight container for later.

Nutritional Information (per donut):

Calories: 110

Fat: 10g

Carbohydrates: 4g

Protein: 5g

Benefits of a Low Carb Diet:

- Supports weight loss
- Helps to regulate blood sugar levels
- Supports heart health
- Promotes increased energy levels
- Supports a healthy digestive system.

Low Carb Classic Donut Recipe

Preparation Time: 10 minutes

Cooking Time: 5 minutes

Total Time: 15 minutes

Ingredients:

- 1 cup almond flour
- 1/4 cup coconut flour
- 1/4 cup sweetener (such as erythritol or stevia)
- 1 tablespoon baking powder
- 1/4 tablespoon salt
- 2 eggs
- 1/4 cup unsweetened almond milk
- 1 tablespoon vanilla extract
- Oil for frying (such as coconut or avocado oil)

Instructions:

1. In a large mixing bowl, whisk together the almond flour, coconut flour, sweetener, baking powder, and salt.

2. Add in the eggs, almond milk, and vanilla extract and mix until well combined.

3. Heat a small amount of oil in a large saucepan over medium heat.

4. Using a cookie scoop or spoon, drop the batter into the hot oil in 2-tablespoon portions.

5. Fry the donuts until golden brown, about 2-3 minutes per side.

6. Remove from the oil and drain on a paper towel-lined plate.

7. Serve immediately, or allow to cool and store in an airtight container for later.

Nutritional Information (per donut):

Calories: 110

Fat: 10g

Carbohydrates: 4g

Protein: 5g

Benefits of a Low Carb Diet:

- Supports weight loss
- Helps to regulate blood sugar levels
- Supports heart health
- Promotes increased energy levels
- Supports a healthy digestive system.

Strawberry Chicken Salad Recipe

Preparation Time: 15 minutes

Cooking Time: 15 minutes

Total Time: 30 minutes

Ingredients:

- 2 boneless, skinless chicken breasts
- Salt and pepper to taste
- 1 cup strawberries, hulled and chopped
- 1/2 cup plain Greek yogurt
- 1/4 cup mayonnaise
- 2 tablespoon honey
- 1/2 tablespoon Dijon mustard
- 1/4 tablespoon salt
- 4 cups mixed greens
- 1/4 cup toasted pecans

Instructions:

1. Season the chicken breasts with salt and pepper and cook until fully cooked through, about 8-10 minutes on each side.
2. Allow the chicken to cool completely before slicing into bite-sized pieces.
3. In a small bowl, whisk together the Greek yogurt, mayonnaise, honey, Dijon mustard, and salt.
4. In a large bowl, mix together the sliced chicken, chopped strawberries, mixed greens, and toasted pecans.
5. Add in the dressing and mix until well combined.
6. Serve immediately, or store in an airtight container in the refrigerator for later.

Nutritional Information (per serving, based on 4 servings):

- Calories: 342
- Fat: 22g
- Carbohydrates: 16g
- Protein: 24g

Benefits of a Diabetic Diet:

- Supports weight management
- Helps regulate blood sugar levels
- Promotes heart health
- Supports healthy blood pressure levels
- Encourages the consumption of nutrient-dense foods.

French Toast with Whole Grain Bread Recipe:

Preparation Time: 5 minutes

Cooking Time: 10 minutes

Total Time: 15 minutes

Ingredients:

- 4 slices of whole grain bread
- 2 eggs
- 1/2 cup unsweetened almond milk
- 1 tablespoon vanilla extract
- 1 tablespoon cinnamon

- 1 tablespoon sweetener (such as erythritol or stevia)
- 1 tablespoon butter or oil for cooking

Instructions:

1. In a shallow dish, whisk together the eggs, almond milk, vanilla extract, cinnamon, and sweetener.
2. Dip each slice of bread into the egg mixture, allowing it to soak for a minute or two on each side.
3. Heat a large skillet over medium heat and add the butter or oil.
4. Cook the French toast for 2-3 minutes on each side, or until golden brown.
5. Serve immediately with your desired toppings, such as fresh berries or syrup.

Nutritional Information (per serving, based on 4 servings): Calories: 174 Fat: 9g Carbohydrates: 18g Protein: 9g

Benefits of a Diabetic Diet:

- Supports weight management
- Helps regulate blood sugar levels
- Promotes heart health
- Supports healthy blood pressure levels
- Encourages the consumption of nutrient-dense foods.

Salmon Burgers Recipe:

Preparation Time: 10 minutes

Cooking Time: 10 minutes

Total Time: 20 minutes

Ingredients:

- 1 lb salmon, skin removed and chopped
- 1/4 cup red onion, finely chopped
- 1/4 cup fresh parsley, chopped
- 2 tablespoon Dijon mustard
- 1 egg
- 1/2 tablespoon salt
- 1/4 tablespoon black pepper
- 2 tablespoon olive oil for cooking
- 4 whole grain buns
- Optional toppings: lettuce, tomato, avocado, etc.

Instructions:

1. In a large bowl, mix together the chopped salmon, red onion, parsley, Dijon mustard, egg, salt, and pepper.
2. Divide the mixture into 4 equal portions and form into patties.
3. Heat a large skillet over medium heat and add the olive oil.
4. Cook the salmon burgers for 4-5 minutes on each side, or until fully cooked through.

5. Serve on whole grain buns with your desired toppings.

Nutritional Information (per serving, based on 4 servings): Calories: 368 Fat: 25g Carbohydrates: 14g Protein: 25g

Benefits of a Diabetic Diet:

- Supports weight management
- Helps regulate blood sugar levels
- Promotes heart health
- Supports healthy blood pressure levels
- Encourages the consumption of nutrient-dense foods.

Open-Faced Tuna Sandwich Recipe:

Preparation Time: 5 minutes

Total Time: 5 minutes

Ingredients:

- 2 cans of water-packed tuna, drained
- 2 tablespoon mayonnaise
- 1 tablespoon Dijon mustard
- 1/4 cup red onion, finely chopped
- 2 tablespoon fresh parsley, chopped
- Salt and pepper, to taste
- 4 slices of whole grain bread, toasted
- Optional toppings: lettuce, tomato, avocado, etc.

Instructions:

1. In a bowl, mix together the tuna, mayonnaise, Dijon mustard, red onion, parsley, salt, and pepper.

2. Toast the slices of whole grain bread.

3. Spread the tuna mixture onto the slices of toasted bread.

4. Add any desired toppings, such as lettuce, tomato, avocado, etc.

5. Serve immediately.

Nutritional Information (per serving, based on 4 servings):

- Calories: 250
- Fat: 10g
- Carbohydrates: 20g
- Protein: 22g

Benefits of a Diabetic Diet:

- Supports weight management
- Helps regulate blood sugar levels
- Promotes heart health

Tomato Basil Pizza Recipe:

Preparation Time: 5 minutes

Baking Time: 10-12 minutes

Total Time: 15-17 minutes

Ingredients:

- 1 pre-made whole grain pizza crust
- 1 cup tomato sauce
- 1 cup shredded mozzarella cheese

- 1/4 cup fresh basil leaves, chopped
- Salt and pepper, to taste
- Optional toppings: diced tomatoes, red onion, mushrooms, etc.

Instructions:

1. Preheat your oven to 450°F (230°C).
2. Place the pizza crust on a baking sheet or pizza stone.
3. Spread the tomato sauce evenly over the crust.
4. Sprinkle the mozzarella cheese over the sauce.
5. Add the chopped basil leaves, salt, and pepper to taste.
6. Add any desired toppings.
7. Bake for 10-12 minutes, or until the cheese is melted and the crust is golden brown.
8. Serve hot.

Nutritional Information (per serving, based on 4 servings):

- Calories: 340
- Fat: 11g
- Carbohydrates: 40g
- Protein: 17g

Benefits of a Diabetic Diet:

- Supports weight management
- Helps regulate blood sugar levels
- Promotes heart health
- Supports healthy blood pressure levels

- Encourages the consumption of nutrient-dense foods.

Southwestern Popcorn Recipe:

Preparation Time: 5 minutes

Total Time: 5 minutes

Ingredients:

- 6 cups popped popcorn
- 1 tablespoon chili powder
- 1 tablespoon paprika
- 1 tablespoon cumin
- 1 tablespoon garlic powder
- 1 tablespoon dried oregano
- 1/2 tablespoon salt
- 1 tablespoon olive oil
- Optional toppings: cheddar cheese, lime juice, chopped cilantro, etc.

Instructions:

1. In a large bowl, mix together the popped popcorn, chili powder, paprika, cumin, garlic powder, oregano, salt, and olive oil.
2. Toss the popcorn mixture until all of the kernels are evenly coated with the spices.
3. Add any desired toppings, such as cheddar cheese, lime juice, or chopped cilantro.
4. Serve immediately.

Nutritional Information (per serving, based on 4 servings): Calories: 120 Fat: 7g Carbohydrates: 13g Protein: 3g

Benefits of a Diabetic Diet:

- Supports weight management
- Helps regulate blood sugar levels
- Promotes heart health
- Supports healthy blood pressure levels
- Encourages the consumption of nutrient-dense foods.

Club Wrap Recipe:

Preparation Time: 5 minutes

Total Time: 5 minutes

Ingredients:

- 4 whole grain wraps
- 8 oz cooked, sliced turkey breast
- 4 slices cooked bacon
- 4 slices reduced-fat cheddar cheese
- 4 large lettuce leaves
- 1 medium tomato, sliced
- 2 tablespoon mayonnaise
- Salt and pepper, to taste

Instructions:

1. Lay out the whole grain wraps on a flat surface.
2. On each wrap, place 2 oz of sliced turkey, 1 slice of cheese, 1 slice of bacon, 1 lettuce leaf, and 2-3 tomato slices.
3. Spread 1/2 tablespoon of mayonnaise over the ingredients on each wrap.
4. Season with salt and pepper, to taste.
5. Roll up the wraps tightly and secure with toothpicks, if desired.
6. Serve immediately or refrigerate until ready to eat.

Nutritional Information (per serving, based on 4 servings):

- Calories: 360
- Fat: 16g
- Carbohydrates: 26g
- Protein: 31g

Benefits of a Diabetic Diet:

- Supports weight management
- Helps regulate blood sugar levels
- Promotes heart health
- Supports healthy blood pressure levels
- Encourages the consumption of nutrient-dense foods.

Grilled Cheese and Pear Sandwich Recipe:

Preparation Time: 5 minutes

Total Time: 10 minutes

Ingredients:

- 4 slices whole grain bread
- 2 oz reduced-fat cheddar cheese, grated
- 1 medium pear, thinly sliced
- 1 tablespoon unsalted butter
- Salt and pepper, to taste

Instructions:

1. Preheat a non-stick pan over medium heat.
2. Lay out the slices of whole grain bread on a flat surface.
3. On 2 of the slices, evenly distribute the grated cheese.
4. Add the sliced pear on top of the cheese.
5. Top the pear with the remaining slices of bread, making 2 sandwiches.
6. Spread 1/2 tablespoons. of unsalted butter over the outside of each sandwich.
7. Place the sandwiches in the pan and cook until golden brown on both sides, about 4-5 minutes per side.
8. Remove the sandwiches from the pan and cut in half, if desired.
9. Serve immediately.

Nutritional Information (per serving, based on 2 servings):

Calories: 300

Fat: 14g

Carbohydrates: 33g

Protein: 14g

Benefits of a Diabetic Diet:

- Supports weight management
- Helps regulate blood sugar levels
- Promotes heart health
- Supports healthy blood pressure levels
- Encourages the consumption of nutrient-dense foods.

Low Carb Pancakes Recipe

Preparation Time: 10 minutes

Cooking Time: 10 minutes

Servings: 2

Ingredients:

- 1/2 cup almond flour
- 2 tablespoons coconut flour
- 1/2 teaspoon baking powder
- 1/4 teaspoon salt
- 3 large eggs
- 1/4 cup unsweetened almond milk
- 1 tablespoon coconut oil
- 1 teaspoon vanilla extract
- Butter or coconut oil for cooking

Instructions:

1. In a medium mixing bowl, whisk together the almond flour, coconut flour, baking powder, and salt.

2. In a separate bowl, beat the eggs and add the almond milk, coconut oil, and vanilla extract.

3. Combine the dry and wet ingredients until well mixed.

4. Heat a non-stick pan over medium heat and add a small amount of butter or coconut oil.

5. Pour 1/4 cup of batter onto the pan for each pancake and cook until small bubbles form on the surface, then flip and cook for another minute.

6. Repeat until all the batter is used up.

7. Serve with your favorite low-carb syrup or toppings.

Nutritional Information (per serving):

- Calories: 325
- Fat: 28g
- Protein: 12g
- Total Carbohydrates: 11g
- Fiber: 5g
- Net Carbs: 6g

Benefits of a Low-Carb Diet: A low-carb diet helps in controlling blood sugar levels and can be beneficial for children with type 1. It also promotes weight loss by reducing insulin resistance and increasing satiety. Additionally, low-carb diets have been shown to improve cholesterol levels, reducing the risk of heart disease.

Sesame Oatcakes Recipe

Preparation Time: 10 minutes

Cooking Time: 15 minutes

Servings: 8

Ingredients:

- 1 cup rolled oats
- 1/4 cup whole wheat flour
- 2 tablespoons sesame seeds
- 1/2 teaspoon baking powder
- 1/4 teaspoon baking soda
- 1/4 teaspoon salt
- 1/4 cup almond milk
- 1 large egg
- 1 tablespoon olive oil
- Butter or oil for cooking

Instructions:

1. In a medium mixing bowl, whisk together the oats, whole wheat flour, sesame seeds, baking powder, baking soda, and salt.

2. In a separate bowl, beat the egg and add the almond milk and olive oil.

3. Combine the dry and wet ingredients until well mixed.

4. Heat a non-stick pan over medium heat and add a small amount of butter or oil.

5. Spoon 1/4 cup batter onto the pan for each oatcake and cook until lightly golden on both sides, about 2-3 minutes per side.

6. Repeat until all the batter is used up.

7. Serve warm with your favourite toppings, such as cheese, honey, or jam.

Nutritional Information (per serving):

- Calories: 100
- Fat: 6g
- Protein: 4g
- Total Carbohydrates: 11g
- Fiber: 2g
- Net Carbs: 9g

Benefits of a Low-Glycemic Diet: A low-glycemic diet, which focuses on carbohydrates with a low glycemic index, can help regulate blood sugar levels for children with diabetes. This can prevent rapid spikes in blood sugar and reduce the risk of heart disease, obesity, and other related health problems. In addition, eating a diet low in glycemic load can also aid in weight loss by reducing insulin resistance and promoting satiety.

Chili and Rosemary Nuts Recipe

Preparation Time: 5 minutes

Cooking Time: 15 minutes

Servings: 8

Ingredients:

- 1 cup mixed nuts (almonds, pecans, walnuts, etc.)
- 2 teaspoons olive oil
- 1 teaspoon chili powder
- 1 teaspoon dried rosemary
- 1/2 teaspoon salt

Instructions:

1. Preheat the oven to 350°F (180°C). Line a baking sheet with parchment paper.

2. In a large bowl, mix the nuts with the olive oil, chilli powder, rosemary, and salt until well coated.

3. Spread the nuts in a single layer on the prepared baking sheet.

4. Bake for 10-15 minutes, or until lightly browned and fragrant.

5. Let cool on the baking sheet for 5 minutes, then transfer to a plate to cool completely.

6. Serve as a snack or add to salads, yogurt, or oatmeal for extra crunch and flavor.

Nutritional Information (per serving):

- Calories: 140

- Fat: 14g
- Protein: 5g
- Total Carbohydrates: 5g
- Fiber: 2g
- Net Carbs: 3g

Benefits of a Low-Carb Diet: Nuts are a low-carb and low-glycemic index food, making them a good option for children with diabetes. They are also high in healthy fats, protein, and fiber, which can help regulate blood sugar levels and promote satiety. Eating a diet rich in low-carb, nutrient-dense foods like nuts can help control blood sugar levels and prevent the development of related health problems. Additionally, the addition of chili and rosemary adds flavor and antioxidants to the snack, further improving its nutritional profile.

Rice Crackers with Hummus Recipe

Preparation Time: 10 minutes

Servings: 4

Ingredients:
- 8 rice crackers
- 1/2 cup hummus
- Fresh vegetables, such as carrots, cucumbers, and bell peppers, for dipping

Instructions:
1. Place the rice crackers on a serving plate.
2. Spoon the hummus into a small bowl and place it in the center of the crackers.
3. Arrange the vegetables around the hummus for dipping.
4. Serve and enjoy!

Nutritional Information (per serving, with 2 crackers and 2 tablespoons of hummus):
- Calories: 120
- Fat: 8g
- Protein: 4g
- Total Carbohydrates: 11g
- Fiber: 2g
- Net Carbs: 9g

Benefits of a Low-Carb Diet: Rice crackers and hummus are a low-carb and low-glycemic index snack, making them a good option for children with diabetes. Rice crackers are made from rice flour, which has a lower glycemic index than wheat flour, and hummus is made from chickpeas, which are high in fiber and protein. Eating a diet rich in low-carb, nutrient-dense foods like rice crackers and hummus can help control blood sugar levels and prevent the development of related health problems. Additionally, the addition of fresh vegetables provides a source of vitamins and minerals, further improving the snack's nutritional profile.

Low Carb Avocado Brownies

Preparation Time: 15 minutes **Baking Time**: 30 minutes **Total Time:** 45 minutes Servings: 9

Ingredients:

- 2 ripe avocados, mashed
- 1 cup almond flour
- 1/2 cup unsweetened cocoa powder
- 1/2 cup erythritol or other low-carb sweetener
- 2 eggs
- 1 teaspoon vanilla extract
- 1/2 teaspoon baking powder
- 1/4 teaspoon salt
- 1/2 cup sugar-free chocolate chips (optional)

Instructions:

1. Preheat the oven to 350°F and line a 9x9 inch baking dish with parchment paper.
2. In a large bowl, mix together the mashed avocados, almond flour, cocoa powder, erythritol, eggs, vanilla extract, baking powder, and salt.
3. Fold in the sugar-free chocolate chips, if using.
4. Pour the batter into the prepared baking dish and spread it evenly.
5. Bake for 30 minutes, or until a toothpick inserted into the center comes out clean.
6. Let the brownies cool in the pan for 10 minutes, then transfer to a wire rack to cool completely.
7. Serve and enjoy!

Nutritional Information (per serving):

- Calories: 205
- Fat: 18g
- Carbohydrates: 11g
- Fiber: 7g
- Protein: 5g
- Net Carbohydrates: 4g

Benefits of the Diet:

- Avocados are a great source of healthy monounsaturated fats, fiber, and potassium.
- Almond flour is a gluten-free alternative to regular flour, and is high in protein and fiber.

Celery Boats Filled with Low Fat Cottage Cheese, Tomato, and Ham or Peanut Butter

Preparation Time: 10 minutes

Servings: 4

Ingredients:

- 8 stalks of celery
- 1 cup low-fat cottage cheese
- 1/2 cup diced tomatoes
- 1/2 cup diced ham or 4 tablespoons of peanut butter
- Salt and pepper to taste

Instructions:

1. Wash and dry the celery stalks, then cut each one into 3 to 4 pieces.
2. Spoon the cottage cheese into a bowl and add the diced tomatoes and ham (or peanut butter) and mix

well. Season with salt and pepper to taste.

3. Spoon the mixture into each celery stalk piece, filling it to the top.

4. Serve immediately and enjoy!

Nutritional Information (per serving, with 2 celery boats filled with cottage cheese, tomato, and ham):

- Calories: 80
- Fat: 2g
- Protein: 12g
- Total Carbohydrates: 6g
- Fiber: 1g
- Net Carbs: 5g

Nutritional Information (per serving, with 2 celery boats filled with cottage cheese and peanut butter):

- Calories: 130
- Fat: 9g
- Protein: 8g
- Total Carbohydrates: 8g
- Fiber: 2g
- Net Carbs: 6g

Benefits of a Low-Carb Diet: Celery, low-fat cottage cheese, and ham (or peanut butter) are low-carb and low-glycemic index foods, making them a good option for children with diabetes. Celery is a low-carb, low-calorie vegetable that is high in fiber and helps regulate digestion, while low-fat cottage cheese is a good source of protein and calcium. Ham (or peanut butter) adds protein and healthy fats to the snack. Eating a diet rich in low-carb, nutrient-dense foods like celery boats filled with cottage cheese, tomato, and ham (or peanut butter) can help control blood sugar levels and prevent the development of related health problems.

Barbecue Popcorn

Preparation Time: 10 minutes

Serving: 2 persons

Ingredients:

- 1/2 cup of popcorn kernels
- 1 tablespoon olive oil
- 1 tablespoon smoked paprika
- 1 tablespoon dried oregano
- 1 tablespoon garlic powder
- 1 tablespoon onion powder
- 1 tablespoon brown sugar substitute
- 1 tablespoon salt
- 1/2 tablespoon black pepper

Instructions:

1. Heat the oil in a large saucepan over medium heat.

2. Add the popcorn kernels and cover the pan with a lid.

3. Once the kernels start to pop, shake the pan continuously to avoid burning.

4. Once the popping slows down, remove from heat.

5. In a separate bowl, mix together the smoked paprika, oregano, garlic powder,

onion powder, brown sugar substitute, salt, and black pepper.

6. Toss the popcorn with the spice mixture until well coated.

7. Serve immediately and enjoy.

Nutritional Information per Serving:

- Calories: 110
- Fat: 7g
- Carbohydrates: 11g
- Protein: 2g

Benefits of the Diet:

- Barbecue popcorn is a delicious and healthy snack option for diabetics.

- The use of brown sugar substitute helps to reduce the overall sugar content of the recipe.

- Popcorn is a high fiber food that can help regulate blood sugar levels and promote a feeling of fullness.

- The spices used in this recipe add flavor and nutrients to the snack, making it a healthier alternative to traditional, sugar-filled snacks.

Baked Beans on Whole Grain Toast Recipe

Preparation Time: 10 minutes

Servings: 2

Ingredients:

- 4 slices of whole grain bread
- 1 can of low-sodium baked beans
- Salt and pepper to taste

- Fresh parsley or green onion for garnish (optional)

Instructions:

1. Preheat your oven to 350°F (175°C).

2. Toast the whole grain bread slices in the oven for 5 minutes, until crispy.

3. Meanwhile, heat the baked beans in a saucepan over medium heat until hot, stirring occasionally. Season with salt and pepper to taste.

4. Remove the toasted bread from the oven and place it on a serving plate.

5. Spoon the hot baked beans over each slice of toast.

6. Garnish with fresh parsley or green onion, if desired.

7. Serve and enjoy!

Nutritional Information (per serving, with 2 slices of toast and 1/2 can of baked beans):

- Calories: 300
- Fat: 3g
- Protein: 15g
- Total Carbohydrates: 53g
- Fiber: 8g
- Net Carbs: 45g

Benefits of a Low-Glycemic Index Diet: Whole grain bread and baked beans are low-glycemic index foods, which means they break down slowly and help regulate blood sugar levels. Whole grain bread is a good source of fiber, B vitamins, and minerals, and baked beans are high in fiber and protein. This snack provides a good balance of carbohydrates, fiber, and protein, making it a good option for children with diabetes. Eating a diet rich in low-glycemic index foods can help control blood sugar levels and prevent the development of related health problem

TASTY DIABETIC SOUPS

Carrot and Ginger Soup Recipe

Preparation Time: 20 minutes

Cooking Time: 30 minutes

Servings: 4

Ingredients:

- 1 tablespoon olive oil
- 1 onion, chopped
- 2 cloves garlic, minced
- 2 teaspoons grated fresh ginger
- 4 cups sliced carrots
- 4 cups chicken or vegetable broth
- Salt and pepper to taste
- Fresh parsley or green onion for garnish (optional)

Instructions:

1. Heat the olive oil in a large saucepan over medium heat.

2. Add the chopped onion, minced garlic, and grated ginger. Cook until the onion is translucent, about 5 minutes.

3. Add the sliced carrots and broth to the saucepan. Bring to a boil, then reduce heat and simmer until the carrots are tender, about 20 minutes.

4. Remove the saucepan from heat and let it cool for a few minutes.

5. Use an immersion blender or transfer the soup to a blender and puree until smooth.

6. Season with salt and pepper to taste.

7. Serve the soup hot and garnish with fresh parsley or green onion, if desired.

Nutritional Information (per serving, with 1 cup of soup):

- Calories: 70
- Fat: 4g
- Protein: 2g
- Total Carbohydrates: 10g
- Fiber: 3g
- Net Carbs: 7g

Benefits of a Low-Carb Diet: Carrots and ginger are low-carb, low-glycemic index foods, making them a good option for children with diabetes. Carrots are high in fiber and vitamins A, C, and K, while ginger is known for its anti-inflammatory and antioxidant properties. This soup provides a good balance of fiber, vitamins, and antioxidants, making it a nutritious and filling snack that can help control blood sugar levels and prevent the development of related health problems.

Mixed Roast Vegetable and Mushroom Soup Recipe

Preparation Time: 30 minutes **Cooking Time:** 60 minutes **Servings:** 4

Ingredients:

- 2 tablespoons olive oil
- 1 onion, chopped
- 2 cloves garlic, minced
- 2 cups sliced mushrooms
- 2 cups diced carrots
- 2 cups diced zucchini
- 2 cups diced eggplant
- Salt and pepper to taste
- 4 cups chicken or vegetable broth
- Fresh parsley or green onion for garnish (optional)

Instructions:

1. Preheat your oven to 400°F (200°C).
2. Toss the diced carrots, zucchini, and eggplant with 1 tablespoon of olive oil, salt and pepper to taste.
3. Spread the vegetables in a single layer on a large baking sheet and roast for 30-35 minutes, until tender and lightly browned.
4. Heat the remaining 1 tablespoon of olive oil in a large saucepan over medium heat.
5. Add the chopped onion, minced garlic, and sliced mushrooms to the saucepan. Cook until the onion is translucent, about 5 minutes.
6. Add the roasted vegetables and broth to the saucepan. Bring to a boil, then reduce heat and simmer for 15 minutes.
7. Remove the saucepan from heat and let it cool for a few minutes.
8. Use an immersion blender or transfer the soup to a blender and puree until smooth.
9. Season with salt and pepper to taste.
10. Serve the soup hot and garnish with fresh parsley or green onion, if desired.

Nutritional Information (per serving, with 1 cup of soup):

- Calories: 130
- Fat: 7g
- Protein: 4g
- Total Carbohydrates: 18g
- Fiber: 5g
- Net Carbs: 13g

Benefits of a Low-Carb Diet: Mushrooms, carrots, zucchini, and eggplant are low-carb, low-glycemic index foods, making them a good option for children with diabetes. These vegetables are high in fiber, vitamins, and minerals, and the roasting process brings out their natural sweetness and flavor. This soup provides a good balance of fiber, vitamins, and minerals, making it a nutritious and filling snack that can help control blood sugar levels and prevent the development of related health problems.

White Bean Soup Recipe

Preparation Time: 10 minutes

Cooking Time: 30 minutes

Servings: 4

Ingredients:

- 1 tablespoon olive oil
- 1 onion, chopped
- 2 cloves garlic, minced
- 2 cups chicken or vegetable broth
- 2 cans white beans (such as cannellini or navy), drained and rinsed
- 1 large carrot, diced
- 1 stalk celery, diced
- Salt and pepper to taste
- Fresh parsley or green onion for garnish (optional)

Instructions:

1. Heat the olive oil in a large saucepan over medium heat.
2. Add the chopped onion, minced garlic, diced carrot, and diced celery to the saucepan. Cook until the onion is translucent, about 5 minutes.
3. Add the broth, drained and rinsed white beans to the saucepan. Bring to a boil, then reduce heat and simmer for 15 minutes.
4. Remove the saucepan from heat and let it cool for a few minutes.
5. Use an immersion blender or transfer the soup to a blender and puree until smooth.
6. Season with salt and pepper to taste.
7. Serve the soup hot and garnish with fresh parsley or green onion, if desired.

Nutritional Information (per serving, with 1 cup of soup):

- Calories: 250
- Fat: 4g
- Protein: 13g
- Total Carbohydrates: 38g
- Fiber: 13g
- Net Carbs: 25g

Benefits of a Low-Carb Diet: White beans are low-carb, high-protein, and high-fiber foods, making them a good option for children with diabetes. This soup provides a good balance of fiber, protein, and healthy carbohydrates, making it a nutritious and filling snack that can help control blood sugar levels and prevent the development of related health problems. Additionally, the vegetables used in this soup (onion, garlic, carrot, and celery) are also low-carb and high in fiber, vitamins, and minerals, providing additional health benefits.

Chickpea and Squash Soup Recipe

Preparation Time: 10 minutes

Cooking Time: 30 minutes

Servings: 4

Ingredients:

- 1 tablespoon olive oil
- 1 onion, chopped
- 2 cloves garlic, minced
- 2 cups chicken or vegetable broth
- 1 can chickpeas, drained and rinsed
- 1 medium butternut squash, peeled and diced
- Salt and pepper to taste
- Fresh parsley or green onion for garnish (optional)

Instructions:

1. Heat the olive oil in a large saucepan over medium heat.
2. Add the chopped onion and minced garlic to the saucepan. Cook until the onion is translucent, about 5 minutes.
3. Add the broth, chickpeas, and diced squash to the saucepan. Bring to a boil, then reduce heat and simmer for 15 minutes.
4. Remove the saucepan from heat and let it cool for a few minutes.
5. Use an immersion blender or transfer the soup to a blender and puree until smooth.
6. Season with salt and pepper to taste.
7. Serve the soup hot and garnish with fresh parsley or green onion, if desired.

Nutritional Information (per serving, with 1 cup of soup):

- Calories: 300
- Fat: 7g
- Protein: 11g
- Total Carbohydrates: 48g
- Fiber: 11g
- Net Carbs: 37g

Benefits of a Low-Carb Diet: Chickpeas and butternut squash are low-carb, high-protein, and high-fiber foods, making them a good option for children with diabetes. This soup provides a good balance of fiber, protein, and healthy carbohydrates, making it a nutritious and filling snack that can help control blood sugar levels and prevent the development of related health problems. Additionally, the vegetables used in this soup (onion and garlic) are also low-carb and high in fiber, vitamins, and minerals, providing additional health benefits.

Moroccan Chicken and Chickpea Soup Recipe

Preparation Time: 10 minutes

Cooking Time: 30 minutes

Servings: 4

Ingredients:

- 1 tablespoon olive oil
- 1 onion, chopped
- 2 cloves garlic, minced
- 1 teaspoon cumin
- 1 teaspoon paprika
- 1/2 teaspoon coriander
- Salt and pepper to taste
- 2 cups chicken broth
- 1 can chickpeas, drained and rinsed
- 1 cup diced cooked chicken
- 1 cup diced carrots
- 1 cup diced zucchini
- Fresh cilantro for garnish (optional)

Instructions:

1. Heat the olive oil in a large saucepan over medium heat.
2. Add the chopped onion and minced garlic to the saucepan. Cook until the onion is translucent, about 5 minutes.
3. Add the cumin, paprika, coriander, salt, and pepper to the saucepan. Cook for another minute, stirring constantly.
4. Add the chicken broth, chickpeas, chicken, carrots, and zucchini to the saucepan. Bring to a boil, then reduce heat and simmer for 15 minutes.
5. Remove the saucepan from heat and let it cool for a few minutes.
6. Use an immersion blender or transfer the soup to a blender and puree until smooth.
7. Serve the soup hot and garnish with fresh cilantro, if desired.

Nutritional Information (per serving, with 1 cup of soup):

- Calories: 300
- Fat: 9g
- Protein: 21g
- Total Carbohydrates: 32g
- Fiber: 7g
- Net Carbs: 25g

Benefits of a Low-Carb Diet: This soup is a great option for children with diabetes, as it is low in carbohydrates and high in fiber, protein, and healthy fats. The chickpeas and vegetables used in this soup are also high in fiber and vitamins, which can help control blood sugar levels and prevent the development of related health problems. Additionally, the spices used in this soup (cumin, paprika, and coriander) are known for their antioxidant and anti-inflammatory properties, providing additional health benefits.

Red Lentil and Bacon Soup Recipe

Preparation Time: 10 minutes

Cooking Time: 30 minutes

Servings: 4

Ingredients:

- 4 slices of bacon, diced
- 1 onion, chopped
- 2 cloves garlic, minced
- 1 teaspoon cumin
- 1 teaspoon paprika
- Salt and pepper to taste
- 4 cups chicken or vegetable broth
- 1 cup red lentils, rinsed
- 2 carrots, chopped
- 2 stalks celery, chopped
- Fresh parsley for garnish (optional)

Instructions:

1. In a large saucepan, cook the diced bacon over medium heat until crispy. Remove the bacon with a slotted spoon and set aside.

2. In the same saucepan, add the chopped onion and minced garlic to the bacon grease. Cook until the onion is translucent, about 5 minutes.

3. Add the cumin, paprika, salt, and pepper to the saucepan. Cook for another minute, stirring constantly.

4. Add the chicken or vegetable broth, red lentils, chopped carrots, and celery to the saucepan. Bring to a boil, then reduce heat and simmer for 20-25 minutes or until the lentils are tender.

5. Remove the saucepan from heat and let it cool for a few minutes.

6. Use an immersion blender or transfer the soup to a blender and puree until smooth.

7. Serve the soup hot, topped with the reserved bacon and fresh parsley, if desired.

Nutritional Information (per serving, with 1 cup of soup):

- Calories: 300
- Fat: 9g
- Protein: 14g
- Total Carbohydrates: 38g
- Fiber: 9g

- Net Carbs: 29g

Benefits of a Low-Carb Diet: This soup is a great option for children with diabetes, as it is relatively low in carbohydrates and high in fiber and protein. The red lentils used in this soup are high in fiber and provide a source of slow-digesting carbohydrates, which can help regulate blood sugar levels. Additionally, the spices used in this soup (cumin and paprika) are known for their antioxidant and anti-inflammatory properties, providing additional health benefits. The bacon used in this soup is a good source of healthy fats, which can help to improve overall health and prevent the development of related health problems.

FRIENDLY AND DELICIOUS SMOOTHIE RECIPES

Strawberry Banana Protein Smoothie

Preparation Time: 5 minutes **Servings:** 1

Ingredients:

- 1 cup frozen strawberries
- 1 medium ripe banana
- 1 scoop vanilla protein powder
- 1 cup unsweetened almond milk
- 1 teaspoon chia seeds

Instructions:

1. Add the frozen strawberries, ripe banana, vanilla protein powder, unsweetened almond milk, and chia seeds to a blender.

2. Blend until smooth, about 1 minute.

3. Pour into a glass and enjoy immediately.

Nutritional Information (per serving):

- Calories: 280
- Fat: 6g
- Protein: 28g
- Total Carbohydrates: 37g
- Fiber: 10g
- Net Carbs: 27g

Benefits of a Low-Carb Diet: This strawberry banana protein smoothie is a great option for children with diabetes, as it is low in carbohydrates and high in protein. The protein powder used in this recipe provides a source of high-quality protein, which can help to regulate blood sugar levels. The almond milk used in this recipe is a low-carb alternative to traditional dairy milk, making it a good choice for children with diabetes. The chia seeds used in this recipe are a good source of fiber, which can help regulate blood sugar levels. Additionally, the ripe banana used in this recipe is a good source of fiber and vitamins, making it a nutritious ingredient for children with diabetes. The use of frozen strawberries in this recipe can help to add sweetness without adding additional carbohydrates.

Low-carb Smoothie Bowl with Berries Recipe

Preparation Time: 5 minutes **Servings:** 1

Ingredients:

- 1 cup frozen mixed berries (such as strawberries, raspberries, and blackberries)
- 1 medium ripe avocado
- 1 scoop vanilla protein powder
- 1 cup unsweetened almond milk
- 1 tablespoon chia seeds

Instructions:

1. Add the frozen mixed berries, ripe avocado, vanilla protein powder, unsweetened almond milk, and chia seeds to a blender.
2. Blend until smooth, about 1 minute.
3. Pour into a bowl and top with additional fresh berries and chia seeds, if desired.
4. Enjoy immediately.

Nutritional Information (per serving):

- Calories: 380
- Fat: 24g
- Protein: 22g
- Total Carbohydrates: 25g
- Fiber: 15g
- Net Carbs: 10g

Benefits of a Low-Carb Diet: This low-carb smoothie bowl with berries is a great option for children with diabetes, as it is low in carbohydrates and high in healthy fats and protein. The protein powder used in this recipe provides a source of high-quality protein, which can help to regulate blood sugar levels. The almond milk used in this recipe is a low-carb alternative to traditional dairy milk, making it a good choice for children with diabetes. The chia seeds used in this recipe are a good source of fiber, which can help regulate blood sugar levels. Additionally, the ripe avocado used in this recipe is a good source of healthy fats, which can help to regulate blood sugar levels. The use of frozen mixed berries in this recipe can help to add sweetness without adding additional carbohydrates. The added fresh berries on top can also provide additional fiber, vitamins, and antioxidants, making this a nutritious and delicious option for children with diabetes.

Green Smoothie with Avocado and Peanut Butter

Preparation Time: 5 minutes

Servings: 1

Ingredients:

- 1 cup fresh spinach leaves
- 1 medium ripe avocado
- 2 tablespoons all-natural creamy peanut butter

- 1 scoop vanilla protein powder
- 1 cup unsweetened almond milk
- 1 tablespoon chia seeds

Instructions:

1. Add the spinach leaves, ripe avocado, creamy peanut butter, vanilla protein powder, unsweetened almond milk, and chia seeds to a blender.
2. Blend until smooth, about 1 minute.
3. Pour into a glass and enjoy immediately.

Nutritional Information (per serving):

- Calories: 460
- Fat: 33g
- Protein: 22g
- Total Carbohydrates: 25g
- Fiber: 13g
- Net Carbs: 12g

Benefits of a Low-Carb Diet: This green smoothie with avocado and peanut butter is a great option for children with diabetes, as it is low in carbohydrates and high in healthy fats and protein. The protein powder used in this recipe provides a source of high-quality protein, which can help to regulate blood sugar levels. The almond milk used in this recipe is a low-carb alternative to traditional dairy milk, making it a good choice for children with diabetes. The chia seeds used in this recipe are a good source of fiber, which can help

regulate blood sugar levels. Additionally, the ripe avocado used in this recipe is a good source of healthy fats, which can help to regulate blood sugar levels. The creamy peanut butter used in this recipe provides a source of healthy fats and protein, making it a nutritious and delicious addition to this smoothie. The spinach leaves used in this recipe can provide additional fiber, vitamins, and antioxidants, making this a nutritious and delicious option for children with diabetes.

Chocolate Avocado Smoothie with Peanut Butter

Preparation Time: 5 minutes

Servings: 1

Ingredients:

- 1 medium ripe avocado
- 2 tablespoons all-natural creamy peanut butter
- 1 scoop chocolate protein powder
- 1 cup unsweetened almond milk
- 1 tablespoon unsweetened cocoa powder
- 1 tablespoon chia seeds
- 1 teaspoon vanilla extract

Instructions:

1. Add the ripe avocado, creamy peanut butter, chocolate protein powder, unsweetened almond milk, unsweetened cocoa powder, chia

seeds, and vanilla extract to a blender.

2. Blend until smooth, about 1 minute.

3. Pour into a glass and enjoy immediately.

Nutritional Information (per serving):

- Calories: 460

- Fat: 33g

- Protein: 22g

- Total Carbohydrates: 25g

- Fiber: 13g

- Net Carbs: 12g

Benefits of a Low-Carb Diet: This chocolate avocado smoothie with peanut butter is a great option for childrens with diabetes, as it is low in carbohydrates and high in healthy fats and protein. The protein powder used in this recipe provides a source of high-quality protein, which can help to regulate blood sugar levels. The almond milk used in this recipe is a low-carb alternative to traditional dairy milk, making it a good choice for children with diabetes. The chia seeds used in this recipe are a good source of fiber, which can help regulate blood sugar levels. Additionally, the ripe avocado used in this recipe is a good source of healthy fats, which can help to regulate blood sugar levels. The creamy peanut butter used in this recipe provides a source of healthy fats and protein, making it a nutritious and delicious addition to this smoothie. The unsweetened cocoa powder used in this

recipe provides a source of antioxidants and can add a rich, chocolatey flavor to this smoothie. The vanilla extract used in this recipe adds a touch of sweetness and enhances the overall flavor of this smoothie.

Strawberry Basil Smoothie

Preparation Time: 5 minutes

Servings: 1

Ingredients:

- 1 cup frozen strawberries

- 1 handful of fresh basil leaves

- 1 cup of unsweetened almond milk

- 1 scoop of vanilla protein powder (optional)

- 1 teaspoon honey or any natural sweetener (optional)

Instructions:

1. Put the strawberries, basil, almond milk, protein powder (if using), and sweetener (if using) in a blender.

2. Blend until smooth and creamy.

3. Pour the smoothie into a glass and enjoy immediately.

Nutritional Information (per serving): Calories: 125 Fat: 3 g Protein: 7 g Carbohydrates: 21 g Sugar: 12 g Fiber: 5 g

Benefits of the Diet:

- The use of almond milk instead of dairy milk helps to keep the calorie and fat content low.

- The addition of protein powder and avocado can help keep you feeling full for longer.

- Strawberries are a low glycemic index fruit, making it a great choice for people with diabetes who need to keep their blood sugar levels in check.

- Basil is a low-carb herb that can add flavor to the smoothie while also providing antioxidants and anti-inflammatory benefits.

Cinnamon Roll Smoothie

Preparation Time: 5 minutes

Servings: 1

Ingredients:

- 1 cup unsweetened almond milk

- 1 ripe banana

- 1 scoop of vanilla protein powder (optional)

- 1 teaspoon of cinnamon

- 1 teaspoon of vanilla extract

- 1 tablespoon of rolled oats

- 1 teaspoon honey or any natural sweetener (optional)

Instructions:

1. Put the almond milk, banana, protein powder (if using), cinnamon, vanilla extract, rolled oats, and sweetener (if using) in a blender.

2. Blend until smooth and creamy.

3. Pour the smoothie into a glass and enjoy immediately.

Nutritional Information (per serving): Calories: 250 Fat: 4 g Protein: 10 g Carbohydrates: 43 g Sugar: 16 g Fiber: 6 g

Benefits of the Diet:

- The use of almond milk instead of dairy milk helps to keep the calorie and fat content low.

- The addition of protein powder and oats can help keep you feeling full for longer.

- Bananas are a good source of fiber and vitamins, making them a great option for people with diabetes.

- Cinnamon helps regulate blood sugar levels and has anti-inflammatory properties.

Dandelion Smoothie

Preparation Time: 5 minutes

Servings: 2

Ingredients:

- 1 cup unsweetened almond milk

- 1 ripe banana

- 1 scoop of vanilla protein powder (optional)
- 1 cup fresh dandelion greens, washed and chopped
- 1 teaspoon honey or any natural sweetener (optional)
- 1 tablespoon of rolled oats

Instructions:

1. Put the almond milk, banana, protein powder (if using), dandelion greens, sweetener (if using), and rolled oats in a blender.
2. Blend until smooth and creamy.
3. Pour the smoothie into a glass and enjoy immediately.

Nutritional Information (per serving): Calories: 180 Fat: 4 g Protein: 10 g Carbohydrates: 33 g Sugar: 13 g Fiber: 5 g

Benefits of the Diet:

- Dandelion greens are a good source of fiber, vitamins, and minerals and are low in calories.
- The use of almond milk instead of dairy milk helps to keep the calorie and fat content low.
- The addition of protein powder and oats can help keep you feeling full for longer.
- Bananas are a good source of fiber and vitamins, making them a great option for people with diabetes.

Broccoli Apple Smoothie

Preparation Time: 5 minutes

Serving: 2

Ingredients:

- 1 cup chopped broccoli florets
- 1 medium apple, peeled and chopped
- 1/2 medium banana, frozen
- 1/2 cup unsweetened almond milk
- 1 scoop vanilla protein powder
- 1 tablespoon honey or sugar substitute
- 1 tablespoon cinnamon
- 1/4 tablespoon nutmeg
- Ice cubes, as desired

Instructions:

1. Add the broccoli, apple, banana, almond milk, protein powder, honey (or sugar substitute), cinnamon, and nutmeg to a blender.
2. Blend until smooth and creamy, adding more almond milk if necessary.
3. Add a few ice cubes and blend until smooth.
4. Pour the smoothie into a glass and enjoy immediately.

Nutritional Information (per serving):

- Calories: 250

- Carbohydrates: 37g
- Fiber: 7g
- Protein: 21g
- Fat: 5g
- Sodium: 200mg

The **Benefit of the diet:**

- The Broccoli Apple Smoothie is a great option for people with diabetes as it contains a balanced mix of carbohydrates, protein, and healthy fats.

- The protein powder provides a good source of protein which helps to regulate blood sugar levels and keep you feeling full for longer.

- The fiber from the broccoli and apple help to slow down the digestion of carbohydrates and prevent rapid spikes in blood sugar levels.

- This smoothie is low in added sugars, making it a great choice for people with diabetes who need to monitor their sugar intake.

Kale Kiwi Smoothie

Preparation Time: 5 minutes **Servings:** 1

Ingredients:

- 1 cup of chopped kale, stems removed
- 1 kiwi, peeled
- 1/2 banana
- 1/2 cup almond milk
- 1/2 tablespoon honey
- 1 scoop of vanilla protein powder (optional)

Instructions:

1. Wash and chop the kale and kiwi, and peel the banana.

2. Add the chopped kale, kiwi, banana, almond milk, honey and protein powder (if using) to a blender.

3. Blend until smooth, about 1-2 minutes.

4. Pour the smoothie into a glass and enjoy immediately.

Nutritional Information (per serving): Calories: 150 Fat: 3g Carbohydrates: 27g Protein: 8g Fiber: 5g

Benefits of the Diet: This smoothie provides essential vitamins, minerals, and fiber, which can help regulate blood sugar levels for those with diabetes. The almond milk provides a low-fat source of protein and healthy fats, while the kale and kiwi are high in antioxidants that can help improve overall health. Additionally, the use of honey in place of added sugars helps to limit the overall carbohydrate content of the smoothie, making it a suitable option for those following a diabetic diet.

Watercress Smoothie

Preparation Time: 5 minutes

Ingredients:

- 1 cup watercress leaves
- 1 kiwi, peeled
- 1 banana, peeled
- 1/2 cup frozen strawberries
- 1/2 cup almond milk
- 1 tablespoon chia seeds

Instructions:

1. Wash the watercress leaves and pat dry.

2. In a blender, combine the watercress, kiwi, banana, frozen strawberries, almond milk and chia seeds.

3. Blend until smooth.

4. Pour the smoothie into a glass and enjoy immediately.

Nutritional Information: Serving Size: 1 smoothie Calories: 220

Total Fat: 7 g

Saturated Fat: 1 g

Sodium: 150 mg

Total Carbohydrates: 36 g

Dietary Fiber: 8 g

Sugar: 17 g

Protein: 8 g

Benefits of the Diet:

- Watercress is a low-carbohydrate and low-calorie vegetable that is high in vitamins and minerals, including vitamin C, vitamin K, and potassium.

- The chia seeds add extra fiber and protein, making this smoothie a nutritious and filling meal or snack.

- The addition of fruit, such as kiwi and strawberries, adds natural sweetness and flavor, making this smoothie a delicious way to incorporate more greens into your diet.

Beet Greens Smoothie

Preparation Time: 5 minutes

Ingredients:

- 1 large beet greens bunch (leaves and stems)
- 2 medium ripe kiwis
- 1 medium ripe banana
- 1 medium green apple
- 1/2 lemon, juiced
- 1 cup almond milk or water

Instructions:

1. Rinse and chop the beet greens and set aside.

2. Peel the kiwis and chop into small pieces.

3. Peel the banana and chop into small pieces.

4. Core the green apple and chop into small pieces.

5. Add the chopped beet greens, kiwis, banana, green apple, lemon juice, and almond milk or water to a blender.

6. Blend on high speed until the mixture is smooth and well combined, about 1-2 minutes.

7. Pour the smoothie into a glass and serve immediately.

Nutritional Information (per serving, based on 2 servings):

- Calories: 120
- Total Fat: 2g
- Saturated Fat: 0g
- Cholesterol: 0mg
- Sodium: 150mg
- Total Carbohydrates: 27g
- Dietary Fiber: 7g
- Sugars: 14g
- Protein: 3g

Benefits of the Diet:

1. Low in sugar: This smoothie is made with low-glycemic fruits, making it an excellent choice for people with diabetes.

2. High in fiber: The beet greens and kiwi in this smoothie provide a good source of fiber, which helps to regulate blood sugar levels and support digestion.

3. Anti-inflammatory: Beet greens contain antioxidants and anti-inflammatory compounds that help reduce oxidative stress and inflammation in the body.

4. Supports heart health: Beet greens are high in nitrates, which can improve blood flow and lower blood pressure, supporting heart health.

5. Boosts immunity: Kiwis are rich in vitamins C and E, which support a healthy immune system.

Cacao Spinach Smoothie

Preparation Time: 10 minutes

Servings: 1

Ingredients:

- 1 banana
- 1 cup baby spinach
- 1/2 avocado
- 1/2 cup unsweetened almond milk
- 2 tablespoons cacao powder
- 1 teaspoon vanilla extract
- 1 scoop of vanilla protein powder (optional)

Instructions:

1. Blend the banana, baby spinach, avocado, almond milk, cacao

powder, vanilla extract and optional protein powder in a blender until smooth.

2. Pour into a glass and enjoy immediately.

Nutritional Information (per serving):

Calories: 314

Fat: 19 g

Protein: 10 g

Carbohydrates: 34 g

 Fiber: 14 g

Benefit of the diet: This smoothie is a great option for people with diabetes as it is low in sugar and high in healthy fats and fiber. The avocado provides monounsaturated fats, which help to regulate blood sugar levels and keep you feeling full for longer. The spinach provides a source of iron, calcium, and vitamin K, and the cacao powder provides a rich source of antioxidants. The addition of a scoop of protein powder can help to balance out the carbohydrates in the smoothie, making it a more balanced and satisfying meal.

HEALTHY AND FRIENDLY LOW CARB DESSERTS

Healthy Gluten-Free Sugar-Free Carrot Cake Recipe

Preparation Time: 45 minutes

Baking Time: 35 minutes

Total Time: 1 hour 20 minutes

Ingredients:

- 2 cups almond flour
- 2 teaspoons baking powder
- 1 teaspoon ground cinnamon
- 1/2 teaspoon ground ginger
- 1/4 teaspoon ground nutmeg
- 1/4 teaspoon sea salt
- 1 cup grated carrots
- 1/2 cup unsweetened almond milk
- 1/4 cup coconut oil, melted
- 3 eggs
- 1/4 cup erythritol or any low-carb sweetener of your choice
- 1 teaspoon vanilla extract

Instructions:

1. Preheat oven to 350°F (175°C). Grease a 9-inch round cake pan.

2. In a large mixing bowl, combine the almond flour, baking powder, cinnamon, ginger, nutmeg, and salt. Stir well.

3. Add the grated carrots, almond milk, coconut oil, eggs, erythitol, and vanilla extract to the dry mixture. Mix well until smooth.

4. Pour the batter into the prepared cake pan.

5. Bake for 35 minutes or until a toothpick inserted in the center comes out clean.

6. Allow the cake to cool completely before serving. Serve with a dollop of low-fat Greek yogurt or coconut cream.

Nutritional Information (per slice, based on 12 slices):

- Calories: 186 –
- Fat: 17g
- Protein: 6g
- Carbohydrates: 8g
- Fiber: 3g
- Sugar: 3g
- **The benefit of this diet:** This cake is gluten-free and sugar-free, making it a suitable option for those with celiac disease or diabetes. -It is made with almond flour, which is low in carbohydrates and high in healthy fats, protein, and fiber.
- Coconut oil and almond milk provide healthy fats, which can help to regulate blood sugar levels.
- Erythritol is a low-carb sweetener that does not raise blood sugar levels, making it a good option for diabetics.

Sugar-Free Coconut Cream Pie Recipe:

Preparation Time: 40 minutes

Baking Time: 20 minutes

Total Time: 1 hour

Ingredients:

- 1 pre-made gluten-free pie crust
- 1 can of coconut milk
- 1/2 cup of sugar substitute, such as Stevia or Erythritol
- 2 tablespoons of cornstarch
- 1/4 teaspoon of salt
- 3 egg yolks
- 1 teaspoon of vanilla extract
- 1/2 cup of unsweetened coconut flakes
- Whipped cream (optional)

Instructions:

1. Preheat your oven to 375°F.
2. In a medium saucepan, whisk together the coconut milk, sugar substitute, cornstarch, and salt over medium heat.
3. Add in the egg yolks and vanilla extract, and continue whisking until mixture thickens and begins to boil, about 5-7 minutes.
4. Stir in the unsweetened coconut flakes.
5. Pour the mixture into the pre-made pie crust.
6. Bake for 20 minutes or until the filling is set.
7. Let the pie cool to room temperature before serving.
8. Serve with whipped cream if desired.

Nutritional Information (per serving):

- Caloric content: Approximately 250 calories
- Fat content: Approximately 19 grams
- Carbohydrates: Approximately 17 grams
- Protein: Approximately 6 grams

Benefit of the diet: This recipe is designed for those with diabetes who need to control their blood sugar levels. The use of sugar substitutes instead of regular sugar helps to reduce the overall sugar content in the recipe. Additionally, the use of a gluten-free pie crust helps to make this recipe suitable for those with gluten intolerance. The coconut milk and unsweetened coconut flakes provide healthy fats and fiber, while the eggs provide a source of protein. This recipe is a balanced, satisfying dessert option for those with diabetes.

Sugar Free Pineapple Lush Cake

Preparation Time: 45 minutes

Ingredients:

- 1 cup almond flour
- 1/4 cup coconut flour
- 1 tablespoon baking powder
- 1/4 tablespoon salt
- 1/2 cup unsweetened almond milk
- 1/2 cup unsweetened applesauce
- 1/2 cup erythritol or other sugar-free sweetener
- 1 tablespoon vanilla extract
- 2 large eggs
- 1 cup crushed pineapple, drained

Filling:

- 1 package (8 oz) of cream cheese, softened
- 1/4 cup erythritol or other sugar-free sweetener
- 1 tablespoon vanilla extract
- 1 cup whipped cream

Topping:

- Fresh pineapple, chopped

Instructions:

1. Preheat oven to 350°F (175°C).
2. In a large bowl, whisk together almond flour, coconut flour, baking powder, and salt.
3. In another bowl, mix together almond milk, applesauce, erythritol, vanilla extract, and eggs.
4. Add the wet ingredients to the dry ingredients and mix until well combined.
5. Fold in the crushed pineapple.
6. Pour the batter into a greased 9-inch spring form pan.
7. Bake for 25-30 minutes or until a toothpick inserted into the center comes out clean.
8. For the filling, in a large bowl, beat cream cheese until smooth.
9. Add in erythritol and vanilla extract and mix until well combined.
10. Fold in the whipped cream.
11. Spread the filling over the cooled cake.
12. Top with fresh pineapple.

Nutritional Information (per serving):

- Calories: 140
- Total Fat: 11g
- Saturated Fat: 5g
- Cholesterol: 45mg
- Sodium: 130mg
- Total Carbohydrates: 7g
- Dietary Fiber: 3g
- Total Sugars: 3g
- Protein: 6g

Benefit of the diet:

- The use of almond flour and coconut flour provides healthy fats, fiber, and protein while reducing the overall carbohydrate content.
- Erythritol, a sugar-free sweetener, helps keep blood sugar levels stable.
- The addition of fresh pineapple and whipped cream provides a burst of flavor while being low in carbohydrates.

- This dessert is a tasty and healthier alternative to traditional high-carb and high-sugar cakes.

Air-Fryer Crispy Chickpeas

Preparation Time: 10 minutes

Cooking Time: 20 minutes

Serving: 2

Ingredients:

- 1 can of chickpeas, drained and rinsed
- 1 tablespoon olive oil
- Salt and pepper to taste
- 1 tablespoon chili powder (optional)
- 1 tablespoon garlic powder (optional)

Instructions:

1. Preheat the air-fryer to 400°F.
2. In a bowl, mix chickpeas, olive oil, salt, pepper, chili powder, and garlic powder.
3. Spread the chickpeas in a single layer in the air-fryer basket.
4. Cook for 20 minutes, shaking the basket every 5 minutes to make sure the chickpeas cook evenly.
5. Serve hot as a snack or side dish.

Nutritional Information (per serving): Calories: 190 Protein: 10g Carbs: 27g Fat: 7g Fiber: 6g

Benefit of the diet:

- Chickpeas are a low-glycemic index food, which means they won't cause spikes in blood sugar levels.
- They are a good source of plant-based protein, fiber, and iron.

- Olive oil is rich in monounsaturated fatty acids and antioxidants, which may have a protective effect against heart disease.
- Air-frying is a healthier cooking method compared to deep-frying as it uses less oil.

Healthy Homemade Oreos Recipe

Preparation Time: 30 minutes

Cooking Time: 15 minutes

Servings: 18 cookies

Ingredients:

- 1 1/2 cups almond flour
- 1/2 cup cocoa powder
- 1/4 teaspoon salt
- 1/4 teaspoon baking soda
- 1/4 cup erythritol or another sugar-free sweetener
- 1/2 cup unsalted butter, softened
- 1 large egg
- 1 teaspoon vanilla extract
- 2 tablespoons coconut flour
- 1/2 cup sugar-free dark chocolate chips
- 1/4 cup heavy cream

Instructions:

1. Preheat the oven to 350°F and line a baking sheet with parchment paper.
2. In a medium bowl, whisk together the almond flour, cocoa powder, salt, baking soda, and erythritol.
3. In a large bowl, cream together the butter and erythritol with a hand mixer until smooth. Beat in the egg and vanilla extract.

4. Gradually mix in the dry ingredients, and then stir in the coconut flour.

5. Using a cookie scoop or tablespoon, drop the dough onto the prepared baking sheet, 2 inches apart.

6. Bake for 15 minutes or until set. Allow the cookies to cool on the pan for 10 minutes before transferring them to a wire rack to cool completely.

7. In a small saucepan, melt the chocolate chips and heavy cream over low heat, stirring constantly until smooth.

8. Spread a generous amount of the chocolate mixture on the bottom of one cookie and sandwich it with another cookie. Repeat for the remaining cookies.

9. Allow the cookies to set in the refrigerator for 10 minutes.

Nutritional Information (per cookie):

- Calories: 140
- Fat: 14g
- Saturated Fat: 7g
- Cholesterol: 35mg
- Sodium: 70mg
- Carbohydrates: 7g
- Fiber: 3g
- Sugar: 1g
- Protein: 4g

Benefits of the Diet:

- This recipe is low in carbs and sugar, making it a great option for those with diabetes.
- Almond flour and coconut flour are used instead of wheat flour, making it gluten-free.

- The use of sugar-free sweeteners and sugar-free dark chocolate helps to keep the sugar content low.
- The addition of healthy fats from avocado and nuts makes this a satisfying and filling snack.

Lemon Cupcakes Recipe:

Preparation Time:

25 minutes to prepare

20-25 minutes to bake

Ingredients:

- 1 1/2 cups almond flour
- 1/4 cup granulated sugar substitute (such as erythritol)
- 2 teaspoons baking powder
- 1/4 teaspoon salt
- 3 large eggs
- 1/2 cup unsalted butter, melted
- 1/4 cup fresh lemon juice
- 1 tablespoon lemon zest
- 1 teaspoon vanilla extract
- 1/4 cup almond milk
- Optional: lemon frosting or powdered sugar for topping

Instructions:

1. Preheat the oven to 350°F. Line a 12-cup muffin tin with cupcake liners.

2. In a large mixing bowl, whisk together the almond flour, sugar substitute, baking powder, and salt.

3. Add the eggs, melted butter, lemon juice, lemon zest, vanilla extract, and almond

milk to the dry ingredients. Mix until well combined.

4. Fill each cupcake liner about 2/3 full with the batter.

5. Bake for 20-25 minutes or until a toothpick inserted into the center of a cupcake comes out clean.

6. Allow the cupcakes to cool completely before topping with lemon frosting or dusting with powdered sugar.

Nutritional Information (per cupcake without frosting):

- Calories: 215
- Fat: 20g
- Protein: 6g
- Carbs: 8g
- Fiber: 3g

Benefit of the diet:

- This recipe is a healthier alternative for those with diabetes as it uses a sugar substitute and almond flour which are low in carbs and have a lower glycemic index compared to traditional ingredients.

- Lemon is a low-carb fruit that is high in fiber and Vitamin C, making it a great addition to this recipe.

- Almond flour is a good source of healthy fats and protein, helping to keep you satisfied and reducing the risk of overeating.

Snickers Ice Cream

Preparation Time: 20 minutes + 4 hours freezing time Servings: 4

Ingredients:

- 1 cup unsweetened almond milk
- 1 cup heavy cream
- 3 tablespoons erythritol
- 1/2 teaspoon salt
- 2 teaspoons vanilla extract
- 1/2 cup creamy peanut butter
- 3 tablespoons unsweetened cocoa powder
- 1/2 cup chopped sugar-free dark chocolate
- 4 sugar-free snickers bars, chopped

Instructions:

1. In a large bowl, whisk together the almond milk, heavy cream, erythritol, salt, and vanilla extract.

2. In a separate bowl, mix together the peanut butter and cocoa powder until smooth.

3. Stir the peanut butter mixture into the almond milk mixture.

4. Pour the mixture into a freezer-safe container and freeze for 2 hours.

5. Stir in the chopped chocolate and snickers bars.

6. Freeze for another 2 hours, or until the ice cream is firm.

7. Serve and enjoy!

Nutritional Information (per serving): Calories: 350 Fat: 34g Protein: 9g Carbohydrates: 13g Fiber: 4g

Benefits of the Diet:

- Sugar-free: Erythritol is a sugar substitute that does not affect blood sugar levels and is safe for diabetics to consume.

- Low in Carbohydrates: The recipe uses almond milk and heavy cream as the base, which are low in carbohydrates and high in healthy fats.

- High in Protein: The peanut butter and snickers bars provide a good source of protein, which can help keep you feeling full and satisfied.

- Good source of Fiber: The almonds and cocoa powder provide a good source of fiber, which can aid in digestion and help regulate blood sugar levels.

Vegan Cinnamon Rolls

Preparation Time: 35 minutes

Cooking Time: 20-25 minutes

Total Time: 55-60 minutes

Servings: 8 rolls

Ingredients:

- 1 1/2 cups all-purpose flour
- 1 1/2 cups whole wheat flour
- 1/4 cup erythritol
- 1/4 cup coconut sugar
- 2 tablespoon active dry yeast
- 1/2 tablespoon salt
- 1/2 cup warm almond milk
- 2 tablespoon vegan butter, melted
- 1 tablespoon vanilla extract
- 1/4 tablespoon cinnamon

For the filling:

- 1/4 cup vegan butter, melted
- 1/4 cup erythritol
- 1 tablespoon cinnamon

For the icing:

- 1 cup powdered sugar
- 2 tablespoon almond milk
- 1 tablespoon vegan butter
- 1 tablespoon vanilla extract

Instructions:

1. In a large mixing bowl, combine both flours, erythritol, coconut sugar, yeast, and salt.

2. In a separate bowl, mix together warm almond milk, melted vegan butter, vanilla extract.

3. Pour the wet ingredients into the dry ingredients and stir until the dough forms.

4. Turn the dough out onto a lightly floured surface and knead for about 5 minutes.

5. Place the dough in a greased bowl, cover and let it rise for about 10-15 minutes.

6. Preheat the oven to 375°F.

7. Roll out the dough into a large rectangle, about 1/4 inch thick.

8. Spread melted vegan butter over the dough, then sprinkle erythitol, and cinnamon.

9. Roll the dough tightly, starting from the long end.

10. Cut the roll into 1-inch slices and place them in a greased 9-inch round baking pan.

11. Bake for 20-25 minutes or until the edges are golden brown.

12. In a medium bowl, whisk together the ingredients for the icing until smooth.

13. Drizzle the icing over the warm cinnamon rolls.

Nutritional Information (per serving): Calories: 286 Total Fat: 14 g Saturated Fat: 5 g Carbohydrates: 41 g Fiber: 4 g Protein: 6 g

The benefit of this diet: This diabetic-friendly vegan cinnamon roll recipe is made with healthier ingredients such as whole wheat flour and erythritol, which is a low glycemic index sweetener that won't spike your blood sugar levels. It also uses vegan butter and almond milk instead of regular butter and milk, making it a good option for those who are lactose intolerant. Eating a balanced diet with a variety of fruits, vegetables, whole grains, and plant-based proteins can help manage blood sugar levels and prevent diabetes-related complications.

Copycat Girl Scout Samoa Cookies

Preparation Time: 45 minutes Servings: 12 cookies

Ingredients:

- 1 cup almond flour
- 1/4 cup coconut flour
- 1/4 teaspoon baking soda
- 1/4 teaspoon salt
- 1/4 cup coconut oil, melted
- 1/4 cup erythritol or other low-carb sweetener
- 1 teaspoon vanilla extract
- 1/2 cup unsweetened shredded coconut
- 1/2 cup sugar-free dark chocolate chips
- 1 tablespoon coconut cream
- 1 tablespoon unsweetened cocoa powder

Instructions:

1. Preheat oven to 350°F and line a baking sheet with parchment paper.

2. In a large mixing bowl, whisk together the almond flour, coconut flour, baking soda, and salt.

3. Add the melted coconut oil, erythritol or other low-carb sweetener, and vanilla extract to the dry ingredients and mix until a dough forms.

4. Using a cookie scoop or tablespoon, form the dough into 12 balls and place them on the prepared baking sheet.

5. Flatten each ball slightly with the back of a fork. Bake for 10-12 minutes or until the edges are lightly golden.

6. In a small saucepan, melt the sugar-free dark chocolate chips and coconut cream over low heat. Stir until smooth.

7. Dip each cookie halfway into the melted chocolate and place on a sheet of parchment paper to set.

8. In a separate small bowl, mix together the unsweetened shredded coconut and cocoa powder.

9. Sprinkle the coconut mixture over the chocolate on each cookie.

10. Allow the cookies to cool completely and the chocolate to set before serving.

Nutritional Information (per cookie):

-Calories: 130

-Fat: 14g

-Protein: 3g

-Carbohydrates: 5g (Net carbs: 2g)

-Fiber: 3g

Benefits of the Diet:

- Low in carbohydrates and sugar, making it suitable for those with diabetes or other carbohydrate-restrictive diets.

- Made with almond flour and coconut flour, which are high in healthy fats and fiber, making them more filling and helping to regulate blood sugar levels.

- Sweetened with erythitol or other low-carb sweeteners, which do not raise blood sugar levels like traditional sugar.

- Rich in healthy fats from the coconut oil and almond flour, helping to promote satiety and reduce cravings.

Low-Sugar Vanilla Ice Cream Recipe

Preparation Time: 15 minutes + 4 hours of freezing time

Ingredients:

- 1 can (13.5 oz) full-fat coconut milk

- 1 cup unsweetened almond milk

- 2 tablespoon cornstarch

- 1 tablespoon. pure vanilla extract

- 1/3 cup granulated erythritol or other low-carb sweetener

- Pinch of salt

Instructions:

1. In a small bowl, whisk together 2 tablespoons of cornstarch with 1/4 cup of almond milk. Set aside.

2. In a saucepan, whisk together the rest of the almond milk, coconut milk, sweetener, and salt.

3. Heat the mixture over medium heat, stirring continuously, until it begins to steam.

4. Stir in the cornstarch mixture into the saucepan and continue to cook for another 2-3 minutes, stirring continuously until the mixture thickens.

5. Remove from heat and stir in the vanilla extract.

6. Pour the mixture into a container, cover and refrigerate for 2 hours.

7. Pour the chilled mixture into an ice cream maker and churn according to the manufacturer's instructions, usually 20-30 minutes.

8. Transfer the ice cream to a container and freeze for at least 2 hours.

Serving size: 1/2 cup

Nutritional Information:

- Cal: 140

- Fat: 12g

- Carbohydrates: 11g

- Fiber: 0g

- Protein: 2g

- Sugar: 3g

Benefits of the Diet: This low-sugar vanilla ice cream is an excellent alternative for people with diabetes who need to control their sugar intake. The use of low-carb sweetener like erythritol and almond milk instead of regular milk and sugar helps in reducing the carbohydrate and sugar content, making it a more diabetes-friendly dessert option.

Chocolate Avocado Ice Cream Recipe

Preparation Time: 10 minutes + freezing time
Serving Size: 4

Ingredients:

- 2 ripe avocados

- 1/2 cup unsweetened cocoa powder

- 1/2 cup unsweetened almond milk

- 1/4 cup granulated sugar substitute (such as stevia or erythritol)
- 1 tablespoon vanilla extract
- Pinch of salt

Instructions:

1. Pit and scoop out the flesh of the avocados into a blender or food processor.

2. Add the cocoa powder, almond milk, sugar substitute, vanilla extract, and salt to the blender.

3. Blend all the ingredients until smooth and creamy.

4. Pour the mixture into a container and freeze for about 3-4 hours, or until firm.

5. Scoop and serve the ice cream.

Nutritional Information:

- Per serving (1/4 of the recipe): Calories: 150 Fat: 13g Protein: 3g Carbohydrates: 13g Fiber: 7g

Benefit of the diet: This ice cream is a low-sugar, low-carb alternative for those with diabetes. Avocados are a good source of healthy monounsaturated fats and fiber, which can help regulate blood sugar levels. Additionally, the unsweetened cocoa powder provides antioxidants and has been shown to improve insulin sensitivity.

Almond Milk Ice Cream

Preparation Time: 20 minutes (plus freezing time)
Servings: 4-6

Ingredients:

- 2 cups unsweetened almond milk
- 1/2 cup heavy cream

- 3/4 cup erythritol or your preferred sugar substitute
- 1 tablespoon vanilla extract
- 1/4 tablespoon salt
- 1/4 tablespoon xanthan gum
- 2 large eggs
- 1 tablespoon cornstarch

Instructions:

1. In a medium saucepan, combine the almond milk, heavy cream, erythritol, vanilla extract, and salt. Heat over medium heat until the mixture starts to simmer.

2. In a small bowl, whisk the xanthan gum with a small amount of the almond milk mixture until smooth.

3. Whisk the eggs in another bowl, then gradually pour the hot almond milk mixture over the eggs while whisking continuously.

4. Pour the egg mixture back into the saucepan and heat over medium heat, stirring continuously, until the mixture thickens (around 5-7 minutes).

5. Remove from heat and let it cool completely.

6. In a small bowl, mix the cornstarch with 1 tablespoon of water until smooth.

7. Pour the cooled mixture into an ice cream maker and churn according to the manufacturer's instructions.

8. While the ice cream is churning, add the cornstarch mixture and let it churn for an additional minute.

9. Transfer the ice cream into a freezer-safe container and freeze until firm (around 2-4 hours).

Nutritional Information (per serving, based on 6 servings):

- Calories: 147
- Total Fat: 14g
- Saturated Fat: 6g
- Cholesterol: 105mg
- Sodium: 119mg
- Total Carbohydrates: 7g
- Fiber: 0g
- Sugar: 3g
- Protein: 4g

The benefit of this diet:

- This low-sugar, diabetic-friendly ice cream recipe uses almond milk and erythritol, which is a low-glycemic sugar substitute, reducing the risk of spikes in blood sugar levels.
- The heavy cream provides a rich and creamy texture while being lower in carbohydrates compared to traditional ice cream recipes.
- Almond milk is a plant-based alternative to cow's milk, making it a good option for those who are lactose intolerant.

Sugar-Free Coconut & Raspberry Cake Ice Cream

Preparation Time: 20 minutes + 4 hours of freezing time

Ingredients:

- 1 cup unsweetened coconut milk
- 1/2 cup frozen raspberries
- 2 tablespoons almond flour
- 2 tablespoons coconut flour

- 2 tablespoons coconut oil
- 1/4 teaspoon stevia extract
- 1/2 teaspoon vanilla extract
- 1/4 teaspoon salt

Instructions:

1. In a blender, combine the coconut milk, raspberries, almond flour, coconut flour, coconut oil, stevia extract, vanilla extract, and salt.
2. Blend until the mixture is smooth and well combined.
3. Pour the mixture into an ice cream maker and churn according to the manufacturer's instructions.
4. Once the ice cream is the desired consistency, transfer it to a container and freeze for at least 4 hours.

Nutritional Information (per serving): Calories: 150 Fat: 15g Carbohydrates: 6g Protein: 2g Sugar: 2g

Benefits of the Diet:

- The use of coconut milk and coconut oil as a base for the ice cream provides healthy fats and helps to keep blood sugar levels stable.
- The addition of almond flour and coconut flour provides fiber and helps to slow the absorption of carbohydrates.
- The use of stevia extract as a sweetener provides a natural, low-calorie alternative to sugar.
- This recipe is also gluten-free, making it a good option for those with gluten sensitivities.

Sugar Free White Chocolate

Preparation Time: 10 minutes + chilling time

Ingredients:

- 1 cup of sugar-free white chocolate chips
- 2 tablespoon coconut oil
- 1 tablespoon vanilla extract
- 1/8 tablespoon salt

Instructions:

1. In a medium saucepan, heat the sugar-free white chocolate chips, coconut oil, vanilla extract, and salt over low heat, stirring frequently, until fully melted and smooth.

2. Pour the melted mixture into a small silicone mold or an 8x8 inch baking dish lined with parchment paper.

3. Chill the mixture in the fridge for at least 1 hour or until fully set.

4. Once set, remove the white chocolate from the mold or cut into desired shapes.

Nutritional Information (per serving):

- Serving size: 1 piece (approx. 1 inch square)
- Calories: 80
- Fat: 8g
- Carbohydrates: 3g
- Protein: 1g
- Fiber: 0g
- Sugar: 0g

Benefits of the Diet:

- This sugar-free white chocolate recipe is suitable for people with diabetes as it contains no added sugars, which helps to regulate blood sugar levels.

- Coconut oil provides healthy fats that can help improve heart health and boost metabolism.

- Vanilla extract is a natural antioxidant that helps to protect the body against harmful toxins.

Note: This recipe is not intended for childrens with a nut allergy, as it contains coconut oil.

Sugar Free Low Carb Vanilla Pastry Cream Recipe

Preparation Time: 20 minutes

Cooking Time: 10 minutes

Servings: 2

Ingredients:

- 1 cup unsweetened almond milk
- 1 cup heavy cream
- 4 egg yolks
- 1/4 cup granulated erythritol or any other sugar substitute
- 2 tablespoons cornstarch
- 1 teaspoon pure vanilla extract

Instructions:

1. In a saucepan, combine the almond milk and heavy cream and heat over medium heat until it starts to steam.

2. In a separate bowl, whisk the egg yolks, erythritol, cornstarch, and vanilla extract.

3. Gradually add in the hot milk mixture while whisking constantly.

4. Pour the mixture back into the saucepan and cook over medium heat, whisking constantly, until it thickens (around 5-7 minutes).

5. Once the mixture has thickened, remove it from the heat and let it cool.

6. Pour the mixture into a container and cover with plastic wrap, making sure the wrap is touching the surface of the cream to prevent a skin from forming.

7. Chill in the refrigerator for at least 2 hours before using.

Nutritional Information (per serving, based on 8 servings):

- Calories: 129
- Fat: 13g
- Carbohydrates: 3g
- Protein: 3g
- Fiber: 0g

Benefit of the diet: This sugar-free and low-carb pastry cream is a great option for people with diabetes as it does not raise blood sugar levels as traditional pastry cream does. It also provides a good source of healthy fats and protein, making it a more balanced option for those following a low-carb or ketogenic diet. The use of a sugar substitute helps to reduce the overall calorie and sugar content, making it a healthier option for those looking to control their sugar intake.

Sugar-Free Low Calorie Homemade Chocolate Marshmallows Recipe

Preparation Time: 15 minutes

Serving; 2

Ingredients:

- 1/4 cup water
- 1 1/2 tablespoons unflavored gelatin
- 1/2 cup erythritol or a sugar-free sweetener of choice
- 1/4 teaspoon salt
- 1/2 teaspoon vanilla extract

- 1/4 cup unsweetened cocoa powder
- Cooking spray or oil
- Confectioners' sugar or cocoa powder for dusting

Instructions:

1. In a large mixing bowl, combine the water and gelatin. Stir until the gelatin has completely dissolved.

2. In a medium saucepan, heat the erythritol or sugar-free sweetener, salt, vanilla extract, and cocoa powder over medium heat. Stir until the mixture comes to a boil.

3. Pour the hot mixture into the mixing bowl with the gelatin and water. Using a hand mixer or stand mixer, beat the mixture on high for 12-15 minutes or until it has doubled in size and becomes light and fluffy.

4. Lightly grease a 9x9 inch square baking dish with cooking spray or oil. Pour the mixture into the dish and spread evenly.

5. Cover the dish with plastic wrap and refrigerate for 2-3 hours or until set.

6. Once set, remove the marshmallows from the dish and cut into squares. Dust with confectioners' sugar or cocoa powder.

Nutritional Information (per serving): Calories: approximately 80 Fat: approximately 1 g Carbohydrates: approximately 11 g Protein: approximately 4 g

Benefit of the diet: This sugar-free, low calorie homemade chocolate marshmallow recipe is perfect for those with diabetes or those looking to reduce their sugar intake. The use of a sugar-free sweetener and unsweetened cocoa powder helps to keep the calorie count and sugar levels low, making it a healthier option compared to traditional marshmallows. Additionally, the high protein content helps to keep you feeling full for longer, making it a great snack option for those with diabetes.

Sugar-Free Cookies And Cream Crunch Recipe:

Preparation Time: 20 minutes

Serving :2

Ingredients:

- 1 cup almond flour
- 1/4 cup unsweetened cocoa powder
- 1/4 cup erythritol
- 1 tablespoon baking powder
- 1/4 tablespoon salt
- 1 egg
- 1 tablespoon vanilla extract
- 1/4 cup unsalted butter, melted
- 2 tablespoon cream cheese, softened
- 2 oz sugar-free white chocolate chips
- 1/2 cup sugar-free cookies, crushed

Instructions:

1. Preheat oven to 350°F and line a baking sheet with parchment paper.
2. In a large bowl, whisk together the almond flour, cocoa powder, erythritol, baking powder, and salt.
3. In another bowl, beat together the egg, vanilla extract, melted butter, and cream cheese until smooth.
4. Add the dry ingredients to the wet ingredients and stir until a dough forms.
5. Fold in the white chocolate chips and crushed cookies.
6. Using a cookie scoop, drop dough onto the prepared baking sheet, about 2 inches apart.
7. Bake for 12-15 minutes, or until the edges are set and the center is still soft.
8. Let cool for 5 minutes before transferring to a wire rack to cool completely.

Nutritional Information (per serving, based on 2 servings): Calories: 350 Fat: 33 g Carbohydrates: 13 g Protein: 10 g Fiber: 6 g

Benefit of the diet:

- Almond flour is a good source of protein and healthy fats, making it a great alternative to traditional flour.
- Using erythritol as a sweetener instead of sugar helps to keep the carbohydrate content low, making it a good option for those with diabetes.
- The addition of cocoa powder provides antioxidants and anti-inflammatory properties.

Note: This recipe is meant as a treat and should not be relied upon as a staple in a diabetic diet.

Sugar-Free Neapolitan Cake

Preparation Time: 40 minutes **Serving:** 8

Ingredients:

- 1 cup almond flour
- 1/4 cup coconut flour
- 1/4 cup Erythritol
- 1/4 teaspoon salt
- 1/4 teaspoon baking powder
- 4 large eggs
- 1/2 cup unsweetened almond milk

- 1/4 cup coconut oil, melted
- 1 teaspoon vanilla extract
- 1 cup strawberries, mashed
- 1/4 cup cocoa powder
- 2 tablespoons Erythritol
- 1/4 cup unsweetened almond milk

Instructions:

1. Preheat oven to 350°F (180°C). Grease and line a 9-inch (23 cm) cake pan.
2. In a large bowl, combine almond flour, coconut flour, Erythritol, salt, and baking powder.
3. In another bowl, beat the eggs, almond milk, coconut oil, and vanilla extract.
4. Add the egg mixture to the dry ingredients and mix well.
5. Divide the batter into three equal parts and place each part in a separate bowl.
6. In one bowl, add the mashed strawberries and mix. In another bowl, add the cocoa powder and Erythritol and mix. In the last bowl, add the remaining almond milk and mix.
7. Pour each batter into the prepared cake pan, starting with the white batter, then the chocolate batter, and finally the strawberry batter.
8. Bake for 25-30 minutes, or until a toothpick inserted into the center of the cake comes out clean.
9. Let the cake cool completely before slicing and serving.

Nutritional Information (per serving):

- Calories: 180
- Fat: 14g
- Carbohydrates: 8g
- Fiber: 4g
- Protein: 7g
- Net Carbohydrates: 4g

Benefits of the Diet:

- Almond flour and coconut flour are low in carbohydrates and provide healthy fats and fiber.
- Erythritol is a low-calorie sugar substitute that does not affect blood sugar levels.
- The use of coconut oil in the cake provides medium chain triglycerides, which are easily metabolized for energy.
- The addition of strawberries and cocoa powder provides antioxidants and phytochemicals for improved health.

Pumpkin Delight

Preparation Time: 20 minutes

Serving: 2 persons

Ingredients:

- 1 cup of pureed pumpkin
- 1/2 cup of almond flour
- 2 tablespoons of coconut flour
- 1/4 cup of erythritol or stevia
- 2 teaspoons of cinnamon
- 1/2 teaspoon of ginger powder
- 1/2 teaspoon of nutmeg
- 1 teaspoon of baking powder
- 1/2 teaspoon of baking soda
- 1/4 teaspoon of salt
- 2 large eggs
- 1/4 cup of unsweetened almond milk

- 1 teaspoon of vanilla extract

Instructions:

1. Preheat the oven to 350°F.

2. In a large mixing bowl, mix together the pumpkin puree, almond flour, coconut flour, erythritol, cinnamon, ginger, nutmeg, baking powder, baking soda, and salt.

3. In a separate bowl, beat the eggs and then add in the almond milk and vanilla extract. Mix well.

4. Add the wet ingredients to the dry ingredients and mix until well combined.

5. Pour the batter into a greased 8x8 inch baking dish.

6. Bake for 25-30 minutes, or until a toothpick inserted in the center comes out clean.

7. Let it cool before serving.

Nutritional Information (per serving):

- Calories: 230
- Fat: 16 g
- Carbs: 18 g
- Fiber: 5 g
- Protein: 9 g

Benefits of the Diet:

- Pumpkin is a good source of fiber, vitamins, and minerals such as potassium, magnesium, and iron.

- Almond flour is gluten-free and is a good source of healthy fats and protein.

- Coconut flour is a good source of fiber and is low in carbohydrates.

- Using erythritol or stevia as a sweetener instead of sugar helps to reduce the overall sugar and calorie content of the dish.

- This dish provides a balanced amount of nutrients, making it a healthy choice for people with diabetes to enjoy.

No-Bake Peanut Butter Pie

Preparation Time: 30 minutes

Serving: 2 persons

Ingredients:

- 1/2 cup graham cracker crumbs
- 2 tablespoons butter, melted
- 1/2 cup creamy peanut butter
- 1/4 cup powdered erythritol or low-carb sweetener
- 1 cup heavy cream
- 1 tablespoon vanilla extract

Instructions:

1. In a medium mixing bowl, mix the graham cracker crumbs and melted butter until well combined.

2. Press the mixture evenly into the bottom and up the sides of a 9-inch pie dish.

3. In another mixing bowl, beat the peanut butter, erythritol, heavy cream, and vanilla extract together until light and fluffy.

4. Pour the mixture into the graham cracker crust and refrigerate until firm, about 2 hours.

Nutritional Information per serving (1/2 slice):

- Calories: 368
- Fat: 35g
- Carbohydrates: 12g
- Protein: 9g

- Fiber: 2g

Benefits of the Diet:

- The low-carb sweetener used in this recipe helps to keep the overall carbohydrate content of the dish low, making it suitable for childrens with diabetes who need to monitor their carbohydrate intake.

- The high-fat content from the peanut butter and heavy cream in this dish can help to provide a slow and steady release of energy, keeping blood sugar levels stable.

- The addition of fiber from the graham cracker crust can help to regulate digestion and keep you feeling full for longer.

German Chocolate No-Bakes

Preparation Time: 15 minutes

Serving: 2 persons

Ingredients:

- 1 cup almond flour
- 1/4 cup unsweetened cocoa powder
- 1/4 cup unsweetened shredded coconut
- 1/4 cup chopped pecans
- 1/4 cup erythritol or any other sugar substitute
- 1/4 cup coconut oil, melted
- 2 tablespoons unsweetened almond milk
- 1 teaspoon vanilla extract

Instructions:

1. In a medium mixing bowl, combine almond flour, cocoa powder, shredded coconut, chopped pecans, and erythritol.

2. Add in melted coconut oil, almond milk, and vanilla extract. Mix until a dough forms.

3. Using a cookie scoop or tablespoon, shape the dough into 12 balls. Place the balls on a sheet of parchment paper.

4. Place the sheet in the freezer for 30 minutes, or until the no-bakes are set.

5. Serve and enjoy!

Nutritional Information (per serving): Calories: 234 Fat: 24g Protein: 5g Carbohydrates: 10g Fiber: 4g Sugar: 2g

Benefit of the diet: This diabetic-friendly recipe is a healthier alternative to traditional German chocolate no-bakes that are high in sugar. By using a sugar substitute and reducing the amount of sugar, the recipe becomes suitable for people with diabetes. Additionally, the use of almond flour and coconut oil provide healthy fats, making it a well-rounded snack option.

Pecan Brownies

Preparation Time: 25 minutes

Serving: 2 persons

Ingredients:

- 1/2 cup almond flour
- 1/4 cup unsweetened cocoa powder
- 1/4 tablespoon baking powder
- 1/4 tablespoon salt
- 2 tablespoon unsalted butter, melted
- 2 large eggs
- 1/4 cup granulated sugar substitute (e.g. erythritol)
- 1 tablespoon vanilla extract
- 1/2 cup pecans, chopped

Instructions:

1. Preheat the oven to 350°F (180°C). Line an 8x8 inch square baking pan with parchment paper.

2. In a medium mixing bowl, whisk together the almond flour, cocoa powder, baking powder, and salt.

3. In a separate large mixing bowl, beat together the melted butter, eggs, sugar substitute, and vanilla extract.

4. Gradually add the dry ingredients to the wet ingredients and mix until just combined. Stir in the chopped pecans.

5. Pour the batter into the prepared pan and smooth out the top.

6. Bake for 20-22 minutes, or until a toothpick inserted into the center comes out clean.

7. Let the brownies cool in the pan for 10 minutes, then transfer to a wire rack to cool completely.

Nutritional Information (per serving, based on 2 servings):

- Calories: 270
- Fat: 25 g
- Saturated Fat: 8 g
- Cholesterol: 95 mg
- Sodium: 140 mg
- Carbohydrates: 12 g
- Fiber: 3 g
- Sugar: 2 g
- Protein: 8 g

Benefits:

- Using almond flour instead of traditional wheat flour reduces the overall carb content, making this recipe suitable for those following a low-carb or diabetic diet.

- Sugar substitute provides a sweet taste without the negative effects of added sugars.

- Pecans are a good source of healthy unsaturated fats, fiber, and minerals like magnesium and potassium.

Sugar-Free Avocado Hummus Recipe

Preparation Time: 10 minutes

Serving: 2 persons

Ingredients:

- 1 ripe avocado
- 1 can of chickpeas, drained and rinsed
- 2 tablespoons of lemon juice
- 1 clove of garlic, minced
- 2 tablespoons of tahini
- Salt and pepper to taste
- 2 tablespoons of olive oil
- Paprika, for garnish (optional)

Instructions:

1. Cut the avocado in half, remove the pit, and scoop the flesh into a food processor.

2. Add the chickpeas, lemon juice, garlic, tahini, salt, and pepper to the food processor.

3. Pulse until the mixture is smooth and well combined.

4. While the food processor is running, slowly add the olive oil and continue to process until the hummus is creamy and smooth.

5. Serve immediately, or store in an airtight container in the refrigerator for up to 3 days.

6. To serve, top with a sprinkle of paprika and serve with fresh veggies, gluten-free crackers, or as a spread for sandwiches.

Nutritional Information (per serving): Calories: 266 Protein: 8g Carbs: 22g Fat: 18g

Benefit of the diet: This avocado hummus is a great alternative for those following a diabetic-friendly diet as it is low in sugar and carbohydrates. The addition of avocados provides healthy monounsaturated fats, which can help regulate blood sugar levels. Chickpeas are a good source of protein, fiber, and slow-digesting carbohydrates, making them a great addition to a diabetes-friendly diet. The use of lemon juice and tahini adds flavor while keeping the dish low in sugar.

Chocolate-Hazelnut Energy Balls

Preparation Time: 15 minutes

Serving: Makes 12 Energy Balls

Ingredients:

- 1 cup hazelnuts
- 1/4 cup unsweetened cocoa powder
- 1/4 cup almond flour
- 1/4 cup unsweetened vanilla almond milk
- 1/4 cup sugar-free maple syrup
- 2 tablespoons coconut oil, melted
- 1 teaspoon vanilla extract
- 1/8 teaspoon salt

Instructions:

1. Preheat your oven to 350°F (180°C) and line a baking sheet with parchment paper.

2. Roast the hazelnuts for 8-10 minutes, or until golden brown and fragrant.

3. Remove from the oven and let cool for 5 minutes.

4. Transfer the hazelnuts to a food processor and pulse until finely chopped.

5. Add the cocoa powder, almond flour, almond milk, maple syrup, coconut oil, vanilla extract, and salt to the food processor and pulse until a dough forms.

6. Scoop the dough into 12 equal portions and roll into balls.

7. Place the energy balls on the prepared baking sheet and refrigerate for 30 minutes, or until firm.

8. Store the energy balls in an airtight container in the refrigerator for up to one week.

Nutritional Information (per serving):

- Calories: 140
- Fat: 13g
- Carbs: 7g
- Fiber: 3g
- Protein: 3g

Benefits of the Diet:

- These energy balls are a low-carb and low-sugar snack option for diabetics.
- Hazelnuts are a good source of healthy fats, fiber, and protein, which can help regulate blood sugar levels.
- Cocoa powder is high in antioxidants, which can help protect against damage from free radicals.
- Almond flour is a good source of protein and healthy fats, and is also low in carbs.

- The use of almond milk and coconut oil instead of dairy and butter helps reduce the calorie and fat content of the recipe.

Strawberry-Chocolate Greek Yogurt Bark

Preparation Time: 10 minutes

Serving: 2

Ingredients:

- 2 cups of Greek yogurt
- 1/2 cup of chopped strawberries
- 1/4 cup of sugar-free chocolate chips
- 1 tablespoon vanilla extract
- 1 tablespoon sweetener of your choice (stevia, erythritol, etc.)

Instructions:

1. Line a baking sheet with parchment paper and set aside.

2. In a large bowl, mix together the Greek yogurt, vanilla extract and sweetener until well combined.

3. Pour the mixture onto the prepared baking sheet and spread it evenly with a spatula.

4. Top the mixture with chopped strawberries and chocolate chips.

5. Freeze the mixture for 1 hour or until solid.

6. Break the bark into pieces and serve immediately or store in an airtight container in the freezer for later.

Nutritional information (per serving, about 1/2 cup): Calories: 120 Fat: 4 g Protein: 13 g Carbohydrates: 13 g Fiber: 2 g Sugar: 7 g

The benefit of this diet: This recipe is a healthier alternative to traditional ice cream, as it uses Greek yogurt which is high in protein and low in fat and sugar. The use of sugar-free chocolate chips and sweeteners reduces the overall sugar content of the recipe, making it a good choice for diabetics. Additionally, the strawberries in the recipe provide vitamins, minerals, and antioxidants, making it a nutritious and tasty treat.

Super-Seed Snack Bars

Preparation Time: 20 minutes

Serving: 2 persons

Ingredients:

- 1/2 cup rolled oats
- 1/2 cup sunflower seeds
- 1/4 cup pumpkin seeds
- 2 tablespoons sesame seeds
- 2 tablespoons chia seeds
- 1/4 cup almond flour
- 1/4 teaspoon salt
- 1/4 cup maple syrup
- 2 tablespoons coconut oil, melted
- 1 teaspoon vanilla extract

Instructions:

1. Preheat the oven to 350°F (180°C). Line an 8x8 inch baking pan with parchment paper.

2. In a large bowl, combine oats, sunflower seeds, pumpkin seeds, sesame seeds, chia seeds, almond flour, and salt. Stir until well combined.

3. In a small saucepan, heat maple syrup and coconut oil over low heat until melted. Stir in vanilla extract.

4. Pour the syrup mixture into the bowl with the seed mixture and stir until well combined.

5. Transfer the mixture to the prepared baking pan, press down firmly to compact the mixture.

6. Bake for 15-20 minutes or until golden brown. Allow to cool completely in the pan before cutting into bars.

Nutritional Information (per serving):

- Calories: 220
- Fat: 17 g
- Carbs: 16 g
- Fiber: 4 g
- Protein: 6 g

Benefit of the diet: These super-seed snack bars are a great option for those with diabetes because they are high in fiber and healthy fats, which help regulate blood sugar levels and keep you feeling full for longer. The seeds also provide essential vitamins and minerals, including magnesium, which is important for maintaining normal blood glucose levels. Additionally, the use of almond flour and maple syrup instead of regular flour and sugar helps to keep the carbohydrate and sugar content low, making these bars a better option for those with diabetes.

Peach Berry Frozen Dessert

Preparation Time: 30 minutes (plus 4 hours for freezing) **Serving:** 4-6 portions

Ingredients:

- 2 cups sliced peaches (fresh or frozen)
- 1 cup mixed berries (fresh or frozen)
- 1/4 cup granulated sugar substitute (such as erythritol)

- 1 tablespoon lemon juice
- 1 tablespoon vanilla extract
- 1/4 tablespoon salt
- 1 cup heavy cream

Instructions:

1. In a blender or food processor, blend the peaches, mixed berries, sugar substitute, lemon juice, vanilla extract, and salt until smooth.

2. In a large bowl, whisk the heavy cream until stiff peaks form.

3. Gently fold the blended fruit mixture into the whipped cream until well combined.

4. Pour the mixture into a 9x9 inch baking dish, and freeze for 4 hours or until firm.

5. Serve the frozen dessert directly from the freezer.

Nutritional Information (per serving):

- Calories: 120
- Total Fat: 11g
- Saturated Fat: 7g
- Cholesterol: 40mg
- Sodium: 150mg
- Total Carbohydrates: 8g
- Fiber: 1g
- Sugar: 6g
- Protein: 2g

Benefit of the diet: This frozen dessert is a low-carb and low-sugar alternative for those following a diabetic diet. The use of sugar substitute instead of traditional sugar helps to reduce the impact on blood sugar levels. The addition of peaches and mixed berries provide a source of fiber and antioxidants.

Low Sugar Chocolate Pie Recipe

Preparation Time: 30 minutes + chilling time
Serving: 8

Ingredients:

- 1 9-inch pie crust, homemade or store-bought
- 3 oz unsweetened baking chocolate
- 1/2 cup granulated erythritol or other sugar substitute
- 2 tablespoons cornstarch
- 1/4 teaspoon salt
- 1 1/2 cups almond milk
- 2 large eggs
- 1 teaspoon pure vanilla extract
- Whipped cream, for serving (optional)

Instructions:

1. Preheat the oven to 350°F. Place the pie crust in a 9-inch pie dish.
2. In a medium saucepan, melt the chocolate over medium heat, stirring constantly.
3. In a large bowl, whisk together the erythritol, cornstarch, and salt.
4. Gradually add the melted chocolate, whisking until well combined.
5. Stir in the almond milk, eggs, and vanilla extract until well combined.
6. Pour the mixture into the prepared pie crust and smooth the top with a spatula.
7. Bake for 25-30 minutes, or until the filling is set and the crust is lightly golden.
8. Allow the pie to cool completely on a wire rack, then chill in the refrigerator for at least 1 hour.
9. Serve with whipped cream, if desired.

Nutritional Information (per serving, without whipped cream):

- Calories: 200
- Fat: 16 g
- Saturated Fat: 7 g
- Cholesterol: 70 mg
- Sodium: 150 mg
- Carbohydrates: 12 g
- Fiber: 2 g
- Sugar: 4 g
- Protein: 6 g

The benefit of this diet: This dessert is a low sugar alternative for those with diabetes who are looking to control their blood sugar levels. The use of a sugar substitute and almond milk helps to lower the overall sugar content of the dish. Additionally, the high protein and fiber content helps to regulate blood sugar levels and keep you feeling fuller for longer.

Peppermint Chocolate Tart

Preparation Time: 25 minutes

 Serving: 8 persons

Ingredients:

- 1 pre-made pie crust, whole wheat or gluten-free
- 1 cup dark chocolate chips
- 1/2 cup heavy cream
- 1 tablespoon peppermint extract
- 1 tablespoon vanilla extract
- Fresh mint leaves, for garnish (optional)

Instructions:

1. Preheat the oven to 375°F (190°C). Place the pie crust in a 9-inch pie dish.

2. Bake the pie crust in the oven for 10-12 minutes or until golden brown.

3. In a saucepan, heat the heavy cream over medium heat until just boiling.

4. Remove the saucepan from heat and add in the dark chocolate chips, stirring until the chocolate is melted and the mixture is smooth.

5. Stir in the peppermint extract and vanilla extract.

6. Pour the mixture into the prepared pie crust and smooth the top.

7. Chill the pie in the refrigerator for at least 2 hours, or until set.

8. Serve chilled and garnish with fresh mint leaves, if desired.

Nutritional Information (per serving):

- Calories: 260
- Fat: 21g
- Saturated Fat: 13g
- Cholesterol: 35mg
- Sodium: 110mg
- Carbohydrates: 21g
- Fiber: 2g
- Sugar: 9g
- Protein: 3g

Benefit of the diet:

- This dessert is a lower sugar alternative to traditional chocolate tarts, making it a suitable option for diabetics.

- Dark chocolate is a good source of antioxidants, which can help protect against cellular damage.

- The use of whole wheat or gluten-free pie crust adds fiber to the recipe, helping to regulate blood sugar levels.

Mini Berry Cream Pies

Preparation Time: 30 minutes

Serving: 6 mini pies

Ingredients:

- 1 cup almond flour
- 1/4 cup Swerve or other sugar-free sweetener
- 1/4 tablespoon salt
- 1/4 cup melted unsalted butter
- 1/4 cup heavy cream
- 1 tablespoon vanilla extract
- 2 cups mixed berries (such as raspberries, blackberries, and blueberries)
- 2 tablespoon Swerve or other sugar-free sweetener
- 1 tablespoon lemon juice
- 2 tablespoon cornstarch
- 1 cup heavy whipping cream
- 2 tablespoon Swerve or other sugar-free sweetener
- 1 tablespoon vanilla extract

Instructions:

1. Preheat oven to 350°F. Line a 6-cup muffin tin with paper liners.

2. In a medium bowl, mix together the almond flour, 1/4 cup Swerve, salt, melted butter, 1/4 cup heavy cream, and vanilla extract until a dough forms.

3. Press the dough into the bottom and up the sides of the muffin cups. Bake for 10-12 minutes, until lightly golden.

4. Meanwhile, in a medium saucepan, combine the mixed berries, 2 tablespoon Swerve, lemon juice, and cornstarch. Cook over medium heat, stirring frequently, until the berries have broken down and the mixture has thickened, about 5-7 minutes.

5. In a large bowl, beat together the heavy whipping cream, 2 tablespoon Swerve, and vanilla extract until soft peaks form.

6. Spoon the berry mixture into the cooled crusts and top with the whipped cream. Serve immediately or store in the refrigerator until ready to serve.

Nutritional Information (per serving):

- Calories: 380
- Fat: 38g
- Carbs: 11g
- Fiber: 4g
- Protein: 5g

Benefit of the diet: This dessert uses almond flour and sugar-free sweeteners instead of traditional wheat flour and sugar, making it a suitable option for those following a low-carb or diabetic diet. The use of healthy fats from the butter and heavy cream, along with fiber from the berries, can help regulate blood sugar levels and provide sustained energy.

Almond & Pear Rose Tarts

Preparation Time: 30 minutes

Serving: 2

Ingredients:

- 1/2 cup almond flour
- 1/4 cup coconut flour
- 1/4 teaspoon salt
- 1/4 teaspoon baking powder
- 2 tablespoons unsalted butter, softened

- 1/4 cup powdered erythritol or sugar substitute
- 1 egg
- 1/2 teaspoon vanilla extract
- 2 medium pears, sliced
- 2 tablespoons sliced almonds

Instructions:

1. Preheat oven to 350°F.
2. In a medium bowl, mix together the almond flour, coconut flour, salt, and baking powder.
3. In a large bowl, cream together the butter, erythritol, egg, and vanilla extract.
4. Gradually add the dry ingredients to the wet ingredients, mixing until well combined.
5. Divide the mixture between two 4-inch tart pans, pressing the mixture evenly into the bottom and up the sides of each pan.
6. Arrange the pear slices on top of the mixture in a circular pattern, slightly overlapping each other.
7. Sprinkle the sliced almonds on top.
8. Bake for 20-25 minutes or until the edges are golden brown.
9. Let cool for 5 minutes in the pans, then remove and let cool completely on a wire rack.

Nutritional Information (per serving): Calories: 245 Fat: 22g Carbohydrates: 13g Fiber: 4g Protein: 6g

Benefit of the diet: This recipe uses almond flour and coconut flour, which are low in carbohydrates and high in fiber, making it a good option for people with diabetes. The use of sugar substitutes helps keep the sugar levels in check while still providing a sweet taste. The high healthy fat content from the almonds and butter provides a satisfying feeling and helps regulate blood sugar levels.

DINNER RECIPES

Chicken & Spinach Skillet Pasta with Lemon & Parmesan

Preparation Time: 30 minutes

Serving: 2 persons

Ingredients:

- 2 boneless, skinless chicken breasts, cut into small pieces
- Salt and pepper
- 2 tablespoons olive oil
- 3 cloves garlic, minced
- 1 teaspoon dried thyme
- 1/2 teaspoon red pepper flakes
- 1/4 cup chicken broth
- 1/4 cup lemon juice
- 2 cups baby spinach leaves
- 2 ounces whole-grain pasta, cooked according to package instructions
- 2 tablespoons grated parmesan cheese

Instructions:

1. Season chicken pieces with salt and pepper.
2. In a large skillet, heat olive oil over medium-high heat.
3. Add chicken and cook until browned, about 5-7 minutes.
4. Add garlic, thyme, and red pepper flakes and cook for 1 minute.

5. Stir in chicken broth and lemon juice, scraping up any brown bits from the bottom of the pan.

6. Add the baby spinach leaves and cook until wilted, about 2-3 minutes.

7. Stir in the cooked pasta and heat until heated through.

8. Top with grated parmesan cheese.

Nutritional Information (per serving):

- Calories: 400
- Total Fat: 16g
- Saturated Fat: 4g
- Cholesterol: 95mg
- Sodium: 580mg
- Total Carbohydrates: 31g
- Dietary Fiber: 4g
- Sugar: 3g
- Protein: 34g

The **Benefit of the diet:** This dish is a low-carb and low-sugar option for people with diabetes. It is high in protein, fiber, and healthy fats, which can help regulate blood sugar levels. The use of whole-grain pasta and spinach provides a source of vitamins and minerals, promoting overall health. The combination of lemon and parmesan cheese adds flavor to the dish without adding additional sugar.

Classic Sesame Noodles with Chicken Recipe

Preparation Time: 25 minutes

Serving: 2

Ingredients:

- 8 oz. spaghetti
- 1 lb. boneless, skinless chicken breasts, sliced into thin strips
- 3 tablespoon olive oil
- 3 garlic cloves, minced
- 2 tablespoon soy sauce
- 2 tablespoon rice vinegar
- 2 tablespoon sesame oil
- 1 tablespoon honey
- 1 tablespoon cornstarch
- 2 tablespoon water
- 1/4 cup chopped scallions
- 1/4 cup sesame seeds
- Salt and pepper to taste

Instructions:

1. Cook spaghetti according to package instructions until al dente.

2. In a large skillet over medium-high heat, heat olive oil.

3. Add chicken strips to the skillet and cook for 5-7 minutes or until browned.

4. Add garlic to the skillet and cook for 1 minute.

5. In a small bowl, whisk together soy sauce, rice vinegar, sesame oil, honey, cornstarch, and water.

6. Pour the sauce over the chicken in the skillet and stir to combine.

7. Bring to a boil, then reduce heat and let simmer for 2-3 minutes or until the sauce thickens.

8. Drain spaghetti and add it to the skillet with the chicken.

9. Toss the spaghetti and chicken in the sauce to fully coat.

10. Sprinkle sesame seeds, scallions, and salt and pepper over the top.

Nutritional Information (per serving):

- Calories: 727
- Total Fat: 44g
- Saturated Fat: 7g
- Cholesterol: 95mg
- Sodium: 1039mg
- Total Carbohydrates: 56g
- Dietary Fiber: 4g
- Sugar: 10g
- Protein: 32g

Benefits of the Diet:

- The use of olive oil in this recipe instead of butter provides healthy monounsaturated and polyunsaturated fats.

- This dish is relatively low in carbohydrates, making it a suitable option for those following a diabetic diet.

- Sesame oil is a rich source of antioxidants and has anti-inflammatory properties.

- Including lean protein sources, like chicken, in your diet can help regulate blood sugar levels and control appetite.

Sheet-Pan Chili-Lime Salmon with Potatoes & Peppers

Preparation Time: 25 minutes

Serving: 2 persons

Ingredients:

- 2 salmon fillets (6 ounces each)

- 1 large red bell pepper, cut into 1-inch pieces

- 1 large yellow bell pepper, cut into 1-inch pieces

- 1 large russet potato, peeled and cut into 1-inch pieces

- 1 tablespoon olive oil

- 1 teaspoon chili powder

- 1 teaspoon garlic powder

- 1 teaspoon ground cumin

- Salt and pepper to taste

- 2 tablespoons fresh lime juice

Instructions:

1. Preheat the oven to 400°F. Line a sheet pan with parchment paper.

2. In a large bowl, mix together the red and yellow bell peppers, potato, olive oil, chili powder, garlic powder, cumin, salt, and pepper.

3. Arrange the mixture in a single layer on one half of the sheet pan. Place the salmon fillets on the other half of the pan.

4. Bake for 18-20 minutes or until the salmon is cooked through and the vegetables are tender and lightly browned.

5. Squeeze the fresh lime juice over the salmon and vegetables. Serve hot.

Nutritional Information (per serving): Calories: 425 Fat: 18g Protein: 36g Carbohydrates: 32g Sodium: 270mg

The **Benefit of the diet:** This dish is a great option for people with diabetes as it is low in carbohydrates and high in protein. The fiber-rich vegetables and healthy fats from the salmon help to regulate blood sugar levels, while the spices and lime juice add flavor without adding extra sugar. Additionally, the high protein content of the dish can help to reduce hunger and cravings, making it a filling and satisfying meal option.

Grilled Chicken with Farro & Roasted Cauliflower

Preparation Time: 15 minutes **Cooking Time:** 30 minutes

 Serving: 2

Ingredients:

- 2 boneless, skinless chicken breasts

- 1 cup farro

- 1 head of cauliflower, cut into florets

- 1 tablespoon olive oil

- 1 tablespoon chili powder

- 1 tablespoon paprika
- Salt and pepper, to taste
- 2 cloves of garlic, minced
- 2 tablespoon lemon juice
- 2 tablespoon fresh parsley, chopped

Instructions:

1. Preheat your grill or grill pan to medium-high heat.
2. Season the chicken breasts with chili powder, paprika, salt, and pepper.
3. In a pot, cook farro according to package instructions until tender.
4. In a large bowl, mix together cauliflower florets, olive oil, garlic, salt, and pepper.
5. Arrange the seasoned chicken breasts and seasoned cauliflower on a sheet pan and grill for 10-12 minutes on each side, or until the chicken is cooked through and the cauliflower is lightly charred.
6. In a serving platter, arrange the cooked farro, grilled chicken, and roasted cauliflower. Drizzle with lemon juice and sprinkle with parsley.

Nutritional Information (per serving):

- Calories: 550
- Fat: 17g
- Saturated Fat: 3g
- Carbohydrates: 63g
- Fiber: 13g
- Protein: 42g

The **Benefit of the diet:** This dish is a great option for diabetics as it is low in sugar and high in fiber and protein. The fiber from the farro and cauliflower helps to regulate blood sugar levels, while the protein from the chicken helps to keep you feeling full for longer. The use of spices and herbs like chili powder, paprika, garlic, and parsley also add flavor without adding extra sugar.

Marinara Meat Sauce Topped Baked Potato Recipe

Preparation Time: 45 minutes

Ingredients:

- 2 large baking potatoes
- 2 tablespoon olive oil
- Salt and pepper to taste
- 1 lb ground beef or turkey
- 1 cup marinara sauce
- 2 cloves of garlic, minced
- 1/4 tablespoon red pepper flakes (optional)
- Fresh basil leaves for garnish (optional)
- Grated Parmesan cheese for topping (optional)

Instructions:

1. Preheat the oven to 400°F.
2. Scrub and wash the potatoes and pat dry. Prick each potato several times with a fork.
3. Brush the potatoes with olive oil and sprinkle with salt and pepper. Place them on a baking sheet and bake for 30-40 minutes, or until the skin is crispy and the flesh is tender.
4. While the potatoes are baking, heat a large skillet over medium heat. Add the ground beef or turkey and cook until browned, breaking it up into small pieces as it cooks.
5. Stir in the marinara sauce, garlic, and red pepper flakes (if using) and bring to a

simmer. Let the sauce cook for about 10 minutes, until slightly thickened.

6. Once the potatoes are cooked, slice them open and top with the meat sauce. Sprinkle with grated Parmesan cheese and fresh basil leaves, if desired.

Nutritional Information (per serving):

- Calories: 460
- Fat: 19g
- Saturated Fat: 7g
- Cholesterol: 75mg
- Sodium: 620mg
- Carbohydrates: 45g
- Fiber: 5g
- Sugar: 6g
- Protein: 30g

The benefit of this diet: This recipe provides a well-balanced meal with complex carbohydrates from the potatoes, protein from the ground beef or turkey, and healthy fats from the olive oil. The marinara sauce is a good source of lycopene, an antioxidant that is beneficial for heart health. Additionally, the fresh basil leaves add flavor and contain vitamins and minerals that are important for overall health.

Homemade Chicken Ramen Noodle Bowls

Preparation Time: 25 minutes

Serving: 2 persons

Ingredients:

- 2 boneless, skinless chicken breasts
- 4 cups of low-sodium chicken broth
- 2 cloves of garlic, minced
- 1 inch of fresh ginger, grated
- 1 tablespoon of sesame oil
- 2 tablespoons of low-sodium soy sauce
- 1 teaspoon of sriracha sauce
- 2 ounces of ramen noodles
- 2 cups of bok choy, chopped
- 1 carrot, julienned
- 1/4 cup of scallions, chopped
- 1 tablespoon of sesame seeds, toasted

Instructions:

1. Preheat oven to 400°F. Line a baking sheet with aluminum foil and set aside.

2. In a large mixing bowl, combine the chicken breasts with garlic, ginger, sesame oil, and soy sauce. Toss to evenly coat the chicken.

3. Place the chicken breasts on the prepared baking sheet and bake for 18-20 minutes, or until fully cooked.

4. In a large saucepan, heat the chicken broth over medium heat. Add the sriracha sauce and stir to combine.

5. Cook the ramen noodles in a separate pot of boiling water for 2-3 minutes, or until fully cooked. Drain the noodles and add them to the saucepan with the chicken broth.

6. Add the bok choy, carrots, and scallions to the saucepan and cook until the vegetables are tender, about 5 minutes.

7. Divide the ramen noodle mixture between 2 serving bowls.

8. Cut the chicken breasts into thin slices and place on top of the ramen noodle mixture.

9. Sprinkle with toasted sesame seeds and serve.

Nutritional Information (per serving):

- Calories: 365
- Fat: 13g
- Carbohydrates: 33g
- Fiber: 4g
- Protein: 32g

Benefit of the diet: This diabetic-friendly recipe is a low-carb, high-protein meal that helps regulate blood sugar levels and control weight. The use of low-sodium chicken broth, low-sodium soy sauce, and reduced-fat ingredients helps keep the overall calorie count low, while still providing essential vitamins and minerals from the vegetables and chicken. The fiber from the bok choy, carrots, and ramen noodles also aids in digestion and helps control blood sugar levels.

Hearty Chickpea & Spinach Stew Recipe

Preparation Time: 25 minutes **Serving:** 2

Ingredients:

- 1 tablespoon olive oil
- 1 medium onion, diced
- 2 cloves garlic, minced
- 1 medium carrot, diced
- 1 medium celery stalk, diced
- 1 teaspoon ground cumin
- 1 teaspoon ground coriander
- 1/2 teaspoon dried thyme
- 1/4 teaspoon red pepper flakes
- 1 can (14.5 ounces) chickpeas, drained and rinsed
- 1 can (14.5 ounces) diced tomatoes
- 1 cup chicken or vegetable broth
- Salt and black pepper, to taste
- 2 cups packed baby spinach leaves

Instructions:

1. In a large saucepan, heat the olive oil over medium heat. Add the onion, garlic, carrot, and celery, and cook until softened, about 5 minutes.
2. Stir in the cumin, coriander, thyme, and red pepper flakes, and cook for 1 minute.
3. Add the chickpeas, diced tomatoes, and broth to the pan, and bring to a boil.
4. Reduce heat and let simmer for 10 minutes.
5. Season with salt and black pepper to taste.
6. Stir in the spinach leaves and cook until wilted, about 2 minutes.
7. Serve hot with crusty bread or over a bed of cooked quinoa.

Nutritional Information (per serving):

- Calories: 304
- Total Fat: 10g
- Saturated Fat: 1g
- Cholesterol: 0mg
- Sodium: 726mg
- Total Carbohydrates: 45g
- Dietary Fiber: 12g
- Sugar: 7g
- Protein: 12g

Benefit of the diet:

- The use of olive oil as the main source of fat provides healthy monounsaturated fats.

- Chickpeas are high in fiber and protein, making them a filling and nutrient-dense ingredient.
- Spinach is a great source of vitamins A, C, and K, as well as folate and iron.

This Hearty Chickpea & Spinach Stew is a delicious and nutritious meal for people with diabetes, as it is low in sugar and high in fiber, protein, and healthy fats.

Easy Pea & Spinach Carbonara

Preparation Time: 15 minutes

Serving: 2

Ingredients:

- 4 oz whole-grain spaghetti
- 1 cup frozen peas
- 2 cups baby spinach
- 2 eggs
- 1/4 cup grated Parmesan cheese
- 2 cloves garlic, minced
- 2 tablespoon olive oil
- Salt and pepper, to taste

Instructions:

1. Cook spaghetti in a pot of boiling salted water until al dente, according to package instructions.
2. Meanwhile, in a large skillet over medium heat, heat olive oil. Add minced garlic and cook until fragrant, about 1 minute.
3. Add frozen peas to the skillet and cook until they are warmed through, about 2 minutes.
4. Add baby spinach to the skillet and cook until wilted, about 2 minutes.
5. Drain spaghetti and add it to the skillet with the peas and spinach.
6. Beat 2 eggs in a bowl and add them to the skillet with the spaghetti mixture, stirring quickly to coat the pasta evenly.
7. Remove from heat and stir in grated Parmesan cheese. Season with salt and pepper to taste.
8. Serve hot and enjoy your delicious and healthy Easy Pea & Spinach Carbonara.

Nutritional Information (per serving):

- Calories: 462
- Fat: 22g
- Saturated Fat: 5g
- Cholesterol: 186mg
- Sodium: 575mg
- Carbohydrates: 46g
- Fiber: 10g
- Sugar: 4g
- Protein: 25g

Benefit of the diet: This diabetic-friendly recipe is a healthy and delicious alternative to traditional carbonara. The whole-grain spaghetti provides fiber and complex carbohydrates, while the eggs and Parmesan cheese offer high-quality protein. The addition of frozen peas and baby spinach increases the nutrient density of the dish and provides important vitamins and minerals. This dish is also low in added sugars, making it a great option for childrens with diabetes.

Lemon Chicken Pasta Recipe

(Serves 2)

Preparation Time: 25 minutes

Ingredients:

- 2 boneless, skinless chicken breasts, cut into small pieces
- Salt and pepper, to taste
- 1 tablespoon olive oil
- 2 garlic cloves, minced
- 2 tablespoons all-purpose flour
- 1 cup low-fat chicken broth
- 1/2 cup heavy cream
- 1/4 cup grated Parmesan cheese
- 2 tablespoons freshly squeezed lemon juice
- 2 tablespoons chopped fresh parsley
- 8 oz. whole wheat spaghetti, cooked according to package instructions

Instructions:

1. Season the chicken pieces with salt and pepper.
2. In a large skillet, heat the olive oil over medium-high heat. Add the chicken pieces and cook until browned, about 3-5 minutes.
3. Add the minced garlic to the skillet and cook for 1 minute until fragrant.
4. Stir in the flour and cook for 1 minute, until lightly browned.
5. Gradually pour in the chicken broth and heavy cream, whisking constantly.
6. Bring the mixture to a boil and then reduce heat to low.
7. Stir in the grated Parmesan cheese and lemon juice. Simmer for 2-3 minutes, until the sauce has thickened slightly.
8. Stir in the chopped parsley.
9. Serve the chicken mixture over the cooked spaghetti.

Nutritional Information (per serving):

- Calories: 482
- Total Fat: 24g
- Saturated Fat: 11g
- Cholesterol: 116mg
- Sodium: 466mg
- Total Carbohydrates: 39g
- Dietary Fiber: 5g
- Sugar: 3g
- Protein: 34g

The benefit of this diet for people with diabetes is that it features whole grain pasta and a relatively low-fat sauce. The fiber from the whole wheat pasta can help regulate blood sugar levels, and the lean protein from the chicken can help keep you feeling full for longer. Additionally, the lemon juice provides a burst of flavor without adding any additional sugar.

Marinara Meat Sauce Topped Baked Potato Recipe

Preparation Time: 1 hour

Serving: 2

Ingredients:

- 2 large russet potatoes
- 1 lb ground beef
- 1 can (28 oz) of crushed tomatoes
- 1 onion, chopped
- 3 garlic cloves, minced
- 1 teaspoon dried basil
- 1 teaspoon dried oregano
- 1 teaspoon dried thyme
- Salt and pepper, to taste

- 2 tablespoons olive oil
- 2 tablespoons grated parmesan cheese

Instructions:

1. Preheat oven to 400°F. Wash and dry the potatoes and then poke each one a few times with a fork.
2. Bake the potatoes for 50-60 minutes or until tender.
3. While the potatoes are baking, heat olive oil in a large saucepan over medium heat.
4. Add chopped onions and minced garlic and cook until fragrant, about 2-3 minutes.
5. Add ground beef and cook until browned, about 5-7 minutes.
6. Stir in crushed tomatoes, dried basil, dried oregano, dried thyme, salt, and pepper.
7. Reduce heat to low and let the sauce simmer for about 20-30 minutes or until thickened.
8. Once the potatoes are done, slice them open and top each one with marinara sauce.
9. Sprinkle parmesan cheese on top and place back in the oven for 5-7 minutes or until the cheese is melted.
10. Serve hot.

Nutritional Information (per serving):

- Calories: 585
- Total Fat: 24g
- Saturated Fat: 8g
- Cholesterol: 74mg
- Sodium: 831mg
- Total Carbohydrates: 69g
- Dietary Fiber: 7g
- Sugar: 12g
- Protein: 32g

The **Benefit of the diet:**

- This dish is a low-carb option for those with diabetes as potatoes are a good source of carbohydrates.
- The use of lean ground beef and a low-sugar marinara sauce helps to control the amount of sugar in the dish.
- Including vegetables like peppers and onions in the dish adds fiber and nutrients to the meal, which is important for overall health.
- This dish is a good source of protein and healthy fats, making it filling and satisfying.

Hearty Chickpea & Spinach Stew

Preparation Time: 15 minutes

Cooking Time: 30 minutes

Serving: 2 persons

Ingredients:

- 1 tablespoon olive oil
- 1 onion, diced
- 2 cloves garlic, minced
- 1 tablespoon tomato paste
- 1 can (14 oz) chickpeas, drained and rinsed
- 1 cup chicken broth
- 1 tablespoon dried thyme
- 1 tablespoon dried basil
- Salt and pepper to taste
- 2 cups baby spinach leaves
- 1 lemon, juiced

- Grated Parmesan cheese, for serving (optional)

Instructions:

1. Heat the oil in a large skillet over medium heat. Add the onion and cook until soft, about 5 minutes.

2. Add the garlic and cook until fragrant, about 1 minute.

3. Stir in the tomato paste, chickpeas, broth, thyme, basil, salt, and pepper.

4. Bring the mixture to a simmer and cook for 10-15 minutes, until the flavors have melded.

5. Stir in the spinach and cook until wilted, about 2 minutes.

6. Stir in the lemon juice and season with additional salt and pepper to taste.

7. Serve hot with grated Parmesan cheese, if desired.

Nutritional Information (per serving):

- Calories: 251
- Total Fat: 9g
- Saturated Fat: 1g
- Cholesterol: 0mg
- Sodium: 710mg
- Total Carbohydrates: 34g
- Dietary Fiber: 8g
- Sugar: 5g
- Protein: 10g

Benefits of the Diet:

- Chickpeas are a great source of protein and fiber, which can help regulate blood sugar levels.

- Spinach is low in carbohydrates and high in vitamins and minerals, making it a great option for those with diabetes.

- The addition of herbs and spices like thyme and basil can help enhance the flavor of the stew without adding extra sugar or unhealthy fats.

- Lemon juice adds a bright, tangy flavor without adding extra carbohydrates or sugar to the dish.

- This stew is a filling and satisfying meal that is both delicious and healthy, making it a great option for people with diabetes.

Easy Jamaican Jerk Chicken Legs with Cabbage Slaw Recipe:

Preparation Time: 15 minutes **Cooking Time:** 30 minutes **Serving:** 2 persons

Ingredients:

- 4 chicken legs
- 2 tablespoons Jamaican jerk seasoning
- 1 tablespoon olive oil
- 1/2 head of green cabbage, shredded
- 1/2 red onion, sliced
- 1/4 cup white wine vinegar
- 2 tablespoons honey
- Salt and pepper, to taste

Instructions:

1. Preheat the oven to 400°F.
2. In a small bowl, mix together the Jamaican jerk seasoning and olive oil.
3. Place the chicken legs on a baking sheet and brush with the Jamaican jerk mixture.
4. Bake in the oven for 25-30 minutes or until fully cooked.
5. While the chicken is baking, prepare the cabbage slaw. In a large bowl, mix together the shredded cabbage, sliced red onion, white wine vinegar, honey, salt, and pepper.
6. Serve the chicken legs with the cabbage slaw on the side.

Nutritional Information (per serving): Calories: 450 Total Fat: 23g Saturated Fat: 6g Cholesterol: 165mg Sodium: 600mg Total Carbohydrates: 22g Dietary Fiber: 3g Sugars: 17g Protein: 40g

Benefits of the Diet:

- This dish is a great source of protein, which is important for maintaining a healthy blood sugar level.
- The Jamaican jerk seasoning adds flavor to the dish while being low in added sugars and carbs.
- The cabbage slaw adds fiber and nutrients, which can help slow down the digestion and absorption of sugars.
- This dish can be a tasty and nutritious option for people with diabetes who are looking for a low-carb, high-protein meal.

Low-Carb Cauliflower Fried Rice with Shrimp

Preparation Time: 20 minutes

Serving: 2

Ingredients:

- 1 head of cauliflower
- 1 tablespoon of olive oil
- 1/2 small onion, diced
- 2 garlic cloves, minced
- 1/2 cup of frozen peas and carrots
- 1/2 teaspoon of ginger paste
- 1/2 teaspoon of dried thyme
- Salt and pepper, to taste
- 2 tablespoons of low-sodium soy sauce
- 1/2 cup of cooked, peeled and deveined shrimp

Instructions:

1. Cut the cauliflower into small pieces and pulse in a food processor until it resembles rice-like grains.

2. In a large skillet over medium heat, heat the oil and cook the onion, garlic, and ginger until fragrant, about 2 minutes.

3. Add the peas and carrots, thyme, and cauliflower rice and cook until the vegetables are tender and the cauliflower is tender, about 5 minutes.

4. Season the mixture with salt and pepper and stir in the soy sauce.

5. Add the shrimp to the skillet and cook until they are pink and heated through, about 2 minutes.

Nutritional Information (per serving):

- Calories: 230
- Fat: 13g
- Saturated Fat: 2g
- Carbohydrates: 13g
- Fiber: 5g
- Protein: 18g

Benefit of the diet: This low-carb and low-sugar dish is a great option for diabetics as it provides a balanced amount of protein and fiber, which can help regulate blood sugar levels and keep you feeling full for longer. The use of cauliflower instead of regular rice also reduces the overall carbohydrate content of the dish.

Chicken Fajita Stir-Fry

Preparation Time: 20 minutes

Serving: 2

Ingredients:

- 1 lb boneless, skinless chicken breast, cut into thin strips
- 1 red bell pepper, sliced
- 1 yellow bell pepper, sliced
- 1 green bell pepper, sliced
- 1 small onion, sliced
- 1 tablespoon olive oil
- 2 cloves of garlic, minced
- 1 tablespoon chili powder
- 1 tablespoon cumin
- 1 tablespoon paprika
- Salt and pepper, to taste
- Juice of 1 lime
- 2 tablespoon chopped cilantro (optional)

Instructions:

1. In a small bowl, mix together chili powder, cumin, paprika, salt, and pepper. Set aside.

2. Heat olive oil in a large skillet over medium heat.

3. Add sliced onions and garlic, and cook for 2-3 minutes until fragrant.

4. Add sliced bell peppers and cook for another 3-4 minutes until soft.

5. Push the vegetables to the side and add the chicken strips. Sprinkle with the spice mixture. Cook until the chicken is no longer pink, about 5-6 minutes.

6. Add the lime juice and cilantro (if using) and stir to combine.

7. Serve hot with a side of brown rice or quinoa.

Nutritional Information (per serving):

- Calories: 367
- Fat: 17g
- Carbohydrates: 20g
- Protein: 34g
- Fiber: 5g

Benefits of the Diet:

- This dish is low in carbohydrates, making it a great option for those with diabetes.

- The chicken and peppers provide a good source of protein and fiber, which can help regulate blood sugar levels and keep you feeling full.

- The spices used in this dish, such as chili powder and cumin, are rich in antioxidants and have anti-inflammatory properties, which can be beneficial for those with diabetes.

- Olive oil, used in this dish, is a healthy source of monounsaturated fats that can help improve cholesterol levels and control blood sugar.

Ginger Beef Stir-Fry with Peppers Recipe

Preparation Time: 15 minutes

Cooking Time: 10 minutes

Serving: 2

Ingredients:

- 1 lb. flank steak, sliced into thin strips
- 1 red bell pepper, sliced into thin strips
- 1 green bell pepper, sliced into thin strips
- 1 yellow onion, sliced into thin strips
- 2 garlic cloves, minced
- 1 tablespoon grated ginger
- 1 tablespoon cornstarch
- 2 tablespoon olive oil
- Salt and pepper, to taste
- 1 tablespoon. low-sodium soy sauce
- 1 tablespoon rice vinegar

Instructions:

1. In a small bowl, mix together the cornstarch, soy sauce, and rice vinegar.

2. Heat 1 tablespoon of oil in a large non-stick skillet over medium-high heat.

3. Add the steak strips to the skillet and season with salt and pepper. Cook for 2-3 minutes until browned on both sides.

4. Remove the steak from the skillet and set aside.

5. Add the remaining 1 tablespoon of oil to the skillet and add the sliced peppers, onion, garlic, and ginger. Cook for 2-3 minutes until the vegetables are tender.

6. Add the steak back to the skillet and pour in the sauce mixture. Stir until the sauce thickens and coats the steak and vegetables.

7. Serve the stir-fry over a bed of brown rice or cauliflower rice.

Nutritional Information (per serving): Calories: 330 Total Fat: 17g Saturated Fat: 5g Trans Fat: 0g Cholesterol: 85mg Sodium: 480mg Total Carbohydrates: 14g Dietary Fiber: 3g Sugars: 5g Protein: 32g

The benefit of this diet: This recipe is a great option for people with diabetes as it is low in carbohydrates and high in protein. The lean flank steak provides a good source of protein and the vegetables provide fiber, vitamins, and minerals. The use of olive oil for cooking is a healthier fat option compared to other oils. This dish is a satisfying and nutritious meal that can help regulate blood sugar levels.

Apricot-Mustard Pork Tenderloin with Spinach Salad

Preparation Time: 20 minutes

Serving: 2

Ingredients:

- 1 pound pork tenderloin
- 1/4 cup apricot preserves
- 2 tablespoons Dijon mustard
- 2 teaspoons olive oil
- Salt and pepper to taste
- 2 cups baby spinach

- 1/4 cup sliced almonds
- 1/4 cup crumbled feta cheese
- 1 tablespoon lemon juice

Instructions:

1. Preheat the oven to 400°F.

2. In a small bowl, mix together the apricot preserves and mustard.

3. Rub the pork tenderloin with the apricot-mustard mixture, making sure it is evenly coated.

4. Heat the olive oil in a large oven-safe skillet over medium-high heat.

5. Sear the pork tenderloin on all sides until golden brown, about 2-3 minutes per side.

6. Transfer the skillet to the preheated oven and roast for 15-20 minutes, or until the internal temperature reaches 145°F.

7. Remove from oven and let it rest for 5 minutes before slicing.

8. While the pork is resting, mix together the baby spinach, sliced almonds, feta cheese, and lemon juice in a large bowl.

9. Serve the sliced pork tenderloin with the spinach salad.

Nutritional Information (per serving): Calories: 391 Fat: 20g Carbohydrates: 19g Protein: 37g Sodium: 590mg

Benefit of the diet: This diabetic-friendly recipe is a healthy and delicious option for those looking to control their blood sugar levels. The use of apricot preserves and mustard provide a sweet and tangy flavor, while the spinach salad provides a good source of vitamins and minerals. The lean protein from the pork tenderloin helps to regulate blood sugar levels, while the low-carbohydrate content of the dish helps to keep blood sugar levels stable. Additionally, the healthy fats from the almonds and olive oil can help to improve insulin sensitivity.

Sweet & Peppery Flank Steak with Shishitos

Preparation Time: 20 minutes

Cooking Time: 20 minutes

Serving: 2

Ingredients:

- 8 ounces flank steak
- 1 teaspoon salt
- 1 teaspoon black pepper
- 2 teaspoons brown sugar
- 1 teaspoon garlic powder
- 1 teaspoon paprika
- 1 tablespoon olive oil
- 8 ounces shishito peppers

For the Spinach Salad:

- 4 cups fresh spinach
- 1/4 cup cherry tomatoes, halved
- 1/4 cup red onion, thinly sliced
- 1 tablespoon balsamic vinegar
- 1 tablespoon olive oil
- Salt and pepper to taste

Nutritional Information:

- Serving Size: 1
- Calories: 452
- Total Fat: 22g
- Saturated Fat: 5g
- Cholesterol: 111mg
- Sodium: 879mg
- Total Carbohydrates: 13g
- Dietary Fiber: 2g
- Protein: 48g

The **Benefit of the diet:**

This dish is a great option for people with diabetes as it is low in carbohydrates and high in protein. The brown sugar in the steak marinade provides just enough sweetness to satisfy cravings without having a significant impact on blood sugar levels. The use of shishito peppers instead of traditional high-carb sides like rice or potatoes also helps keep the dish low in carbohydrates. The accompanying spinach salad is a great source of fiber and vitamins, making this dish a well-rounded and nutritious option for people with diabetes.

Moroccan Chicken & Tomato Stew Recipe

Preparation Time: 20 minutes

Cooking Time: 30 minutes

Serving: 2

Ingredients:

- 1 pound boneless, skinless chicken breast, cut into bite-sized pieces
- 2 tablespoons olive oil
- 1 large onion, diced
- 3 cloves garlic, minced
- 2 tablespoons tomato paste
- 1 teaspoon cumin
- 1 teaspoon paprika
- 1/2 teaspoon coriander
- 1/2 teaspoon cinnamon
- 1/4 teaspoon cayenne pepper

- 1 (14-ounce) can diced tomatoes
- 1 cup chicken broth
- Salt and pepper to taste
- 1/4 cup chopped fresh cilantro

Instructions:

1. Heat 1 tablespoon of oil in a large skillet over medium-high heat.
2. Add chicken to the skillet and cook until browned on all sides, about 5 minutes. Remove from the skillet and set aside.
3. In the same skillet, add the remaining oil and the onions. Cook until the onions are soft and translucent, about 5 minutes.
4. Add garlic to the skillet and cook for another minute.
5. Add tomato paste, cumin, paprika, coriander, cinnamon, and cayenne pepper to the skillet and stir to combine.
6. Add the diced tomatoes and chicken broth to the skillet and stir to combine.
7. Return the chicken to the skillet and bring the mixture to a boil.
8. Reduce the heat to low and let the stew simmer for 20 minutes or until the chicken is cooked through and the sauce has thickened.
9. Season with salt and pepper to taste.
10. Serve the stew over rice or with crusty bread and top with chopped cilantro.

Nutritional Information (per serving):

- Calories: 393
- Fat: 16.3g
- Saturated Fat: 3g
- Cholesterol: 99mg
- Sodium: 624mg
- Carbohydrates: 17.8g
- Fiber: 4.1g
- Sugar: 8.8g
- Protein: 42.6g

Benefits of the Diet:

- The chicken provides lean protein, which is essential for maintaining and repairing body tissues.
- Olive oil is a good source of healthy fats and helps to reduce inflammation.
- The spices used in the recipe, such as cumin, paprika, and cinnamon, contain antioxidants that help to protect against cellular damage.
- The cilantro provides a good source of vitamins and minerals, including vitamin K, vitamin A, and potassium.
- The combination of protein, healthy fats, and fiber from the ingredients in this dish will help to regulate blood sugar levels, making it an excellent option for childrens with diabetes.

Diabetic Recipe: Herby Mediterranean Fish with Wilted Greens & Mushrooms

Serving: 2

Preparation Time: 30 minutes

Ingredients:

- 2 (4 oz) white fish fillets, such as cod or halibut
- Salt and pepper, to taste
- 1 tablespoon olive oil
- 1 large garlic clove, minced
- 1 large shallot, minced

- 2 cups chopped mushrooms
- 1 tablespoon dried oregano
- 1 tablespoon dried thyme
- 1 tablespoon lemon juice
- 1 cup baby spinach leaves
- 1 tablespoon grated Parmesan cheese

Instructions:

1. Season both sides of the fish fillets with salt and pepper.
2. Heat the olive oil in a large skillet over medium heat. Add the garlic and shallot and cook until fragrant, about 1 minute.
3. Add the mushrooms, oregano, and thyme and cook until the mushrooms are tender and the liquid has evaporated, about 5-7 minutes.
4. Add the lemon juice and spinach to the skillet and stir until the spinach is wilted, about 2 minutes.
5. Place the fish fillets in the skillet and cook until just cooked through, about 5-7 minutes.
6. Serve the fish with the wilted greens and mushrooms and top with grated Parmesan cheese.

Nutritional Information (per serving): Calories: 242 Fat: 10.6g Saturated Fat: 2.3g Cholesterol: 70mg Sodium: 243mg Carbohydrates: 7.7g Fiber: 2.1g Sugar: 3.2g Protein: 28g

Benefit of the diet:

- This dish is low in carbohydrates and high in protein, making it a great option for people with diabetes who are trying to regulate their blood sugar levels.
- The use of healthy fats from the olive oil and the addition of fiber-rich vegetables like mushrooms and spinach make this

meal a nutritious option for overall health and wellness.

- The inclusion of herbs like oregano and thyme add flavor without adding extra sugar, making this a delicious and diabetes-friendly meal option.

Chopped Salad with Shrimp, Apples & Pecans

Preparation Time: 15 minutes

Serving: 2 persons

Ingredients:

- 8 oz. cooked, peeled, and deveined shrimp
- 2 cups mixed greens
- 1 medium red apple, cored and diced
- 1/4 cup pecans, chopped
- 2 tablespoon red onion, diced
- 2 tablespoon dried cranberries
- 2 tablespoon low-fat vinaigrette dressing

Instructions:

1. In a large bowl, combine the mixed greens, apple, pecans, red onion, and dried cranberries.
2. Add the cooked shrimp to the bowl and gently toss to combine.
3. Drizzle with the vinaigrette dressing and gently toss to evenly distribute.
4. Serve immediately, dividing the salad evenly between two plates.

Nutritional Information (per serving): Calories: 275 Fat: 13g Protein: 26g Carbohydrates: 18g Fiber: 4g

Benefit of the diet:

- The use of mixed greens, apples, and pecans provides a source of fiber, vitamins, and minerals that support overall health and help regulate blood sugar levels.

- The addition of shrimp provides a lean source of protein that can help to control hunger and maintain blood sugar levels.

- The use of low-fat vinaigrette dressing helps to limit the amount of added fat and calories in the dish, making it a healthier choice for those with diabetes.

Mushroom & Tofu Stir-Fry

Preparation Time: 20 minutes

Serving: 2

Ingredients:

- 1 block of firm tofu, drained and pressed
- 2 cups sliced mixed mushrooms (such as shiitake and cremini)
- 1 red bell pepper, thinly sliced
- 2 garlic cloves, minced
- 1 tablespoon fresh ginger, grated
- 2 tablespoon low-sodium soy sauce
- 1 tablespoon sesame oil
- 1 tablespoon cornstarch
- 2 scallions, sliced (optional)
- Salt and pepper, to taste
- Steamed brown rice, for serving

Instructions:

1. Cut the tofu into small cubes and set aside.
2. In a large skillet over medium heat, heat the sesame oil.
3. Add the garlic and ginger and cook for 1 minute, stirring constantly.
4. Add the mushrooms and red bell pepper to the skillet and cook until softened, about 5 minutes.
5. In a small bowl, whisk together the soy sauce and cornstarch.
6. Add the tofu to the skillet and cook for 2-3 minutes, stirring occasionally.
7. Pour the soy sauce mixture over the tofu and stir to combine.
8. Cook for another 2-3 minutes, until the sauce has thickened.
9. Serve over steamed brown rice, topped with sliced scallions, if desired.

Nutritional Information (per serving):

- Calories: 300
- Carbohydrates: 26 g
- Protein: 20 g
- Fat: 15 g
- Fiber: 3 g

Benefit of the diet:

- This dish is a healthy option for those with diabetes, as it is low in carbohydrates and high in protein.

- The use of sesame oil, ginger, and garlic is beneficial for people with diabetes, as these ingredients have been shown to help regulate blood sugar levels.

- The tofu is a good source of plant-based protein and contains no saturated fat or cholesterol, making it a healthier alternative to meat.

- The mushrooms and red bell pepper provide important vitamins and minerals, including vitamin C and potassium, and help to add variety to the diet.

Shrimp Scampi

Preparation Time: 15 minutes

Serving: 2

Ingredients:

- 1 lb large shrimp, peeled and deveined
- 3 cloves garlic, minced
- 1 tablespoon olive oil
- 2 tablespoon unsalted butter
- 1 lemon, juiced
- 1/4 cup white wine
- 1/4 tablespoon red pepper flakes
- Salt and black pepper, to taste
- 1/4 cup fresh parsley, chopped
- 2 tablespoon grated Parmesan cheese
- 2 tablespoon chopped walnuts

Instructions:

1. Heat a large skillet over medium heat. Add the olive oil and butter.
2. Once the butter has melted, add the garlic and red pepper flakes and sauté for 30 seconds.
3. Add the shrimp and cook until pink, about 2-3 minutes on each side.
4. Add the white wine and lemon juice, bring to a simmer and cook for an additional 2 minutes.
5. Season with salt and black pepper to taste.
6. Stir in the parsley, Parmesan cheese, and chopped walnuts.

7. Serve hot over a bed of cooked whole-grain pasta or zucchini noodles.

Nutritional Information (per serving):

- Calories: 460
- Total Fat: 29g
- Saturated Fat: 11g
- Cholesterol: 400mg
- Sodium: 690mg
- Total Carbohydrates: 8g
- Dietary Fiber: 1g
- Sugars: 2g
- Protein: 44g

Benefits of the Diet:

- The dish is low in carbohydrates, making it a good option for diabetics who need to manage their blood sugar levels.
- The use of whole-grain pasta or zucchini noodles provides a source of complex carbohydrates, fiber, and nutrients.
- The high protein content of the dish helps to keep you full and satisfied for longer periods of time, which can help prevent overeating and weight gain.
- The dish is also a good source of healthy fats, including monounsaturated and polyunsaturated fats, which are beneficial for overall health and heart health.

Rosemary Chicken with Sweet Potatoes

Preparation Time: 30 minutes

Serving: 2

Ingredients:

- 2 boneless, skinless chicken breasts

- 2 medium sweet potatoes, peeled and diced into small pieces
- 3 tablespoon olive oil, divided
- Salt and pepper, to taste
- 1 tablespoon dried rosemary
- 2 cloves garlic, minced
- 1 tablespoon lemon juice
- 1 tablespoon honey

Instructions:

1. Preheat oven to 400°F (200°C).
2. In a large bowl, toss the sweet potato pieces with 2 tablespoons of olive oil, salt, and pepper.
3. Spread the sweet potatoes evenly on a large baking sheet. Roast in the oven for 25 minutes.
4. Meanwhile, in another bowl, mix the rosemary, garlic, lemon juice, honey, and remaining 1 tablespoon of olive oil.
5. Season the chicken breasts with salt and pepper, and then coat them with the rosemary mixture.
6. Once the sweet potatoes have roasted for 25 minutes, add the chicken breasts to the same baking sheet and return to the oven.
7. Bake for an additional 20-25 minutes, or until the chicken is fully cooked and the internal temperature reaches 165°F (74°C).
8. Serve the roasted sweet potatoes and rosemary chicken on a plate and garnish with fresh lemon wedges.

Nutritional Information per **Serving:**

- Calories: 710
- Total Fat: 29g
- Saturated Fat: 4g
- Cholesterol: 165mg
- Sodium: 210mg
- Total Carbohydrates: 64g
- Fiber: 6g
- Sugars: 21g
- Protein: 46g

The **Benefit of the diet:**

- This dish is a good source of protein and fiber, which helps regulate blood sugar levels and keep you full for longer periods of time.
- Sweet potatoes are a good source of complex carbohydrates and vitamins, making them a great alternative to white potatoes for diabetics.
- Rosemary has been shown to have a positive effect on blood sugar levels, making this dish a great choice for people with diabetes.
- The addition of lemon and honey add flavor to the dish without adding excessive amounts of sugar.

DELICIOUS LOW CARB APPETIZER

Olives and Cheese

Preparation Time: 10 minutes **Serving:** 2 persons

Ingredients:

- 1/2 cup of mixed green and black olives, pitted and chopped
- 1/2 cup of cherry tomatoes, chopped
- 1/4 cup of crumbled feta cheese
- 2 tablespoons of extra-virgin olive oil
- 1 tablespoon of freshly squeezed lemon juice
- 1/4 teaspoon of black pepper
- 1/4 teaspoon of dried oregano

Instructions:

1. In a medium-sized mixing bowl, combine the chopped olives, tomatoes, feta cheese, olive oil, lemon juice, black pepper, and dried oregano.
2. Mix everything well to combine.
3. Serve the olives and cheese mixture with crackers, bread, or as a topping for grilled chicken or fish.

Nutritional Information (per serving):

- Calories: 250
- Fat: 24 g
- Saturated Fat: 6 g
- Cholesterol: 20 mg
- Sodium: 540 mg
- Carbohydrates: 7 g
- Fiber: 2 g
- Sugar: 2 g

- Protein: 6 g

The **Benefit of the diet:** Olives and cheese is a healthy and satisfying snack option for people with diabetes. Olives are rich in healthy monounsaturated fats and antioxidants that help regulate blood sugar levels, reduce inflammation, and lower the risk of heart disease. Cheese is a good source of calcium and protein, which helps to maintain healthy bones and muscle mass. This snack is also low in carbohydrates, making it a great option for those who need to manage their blood sugar levels. Additionally, the lemon juice and olive oil add flavor and nutrients, making this snack a well-rounded option for people with diabetes.

Garlic Cheese Loaf Recipe

Preparation Time: 15 minutes

Cooking Time: 30 minutes

Servings: 2

Ingredients:

- 2 slices of whole grain bread
- 2 cloves of garlic, minced
- 1/4 cup of shredded mozzarella cheese
- 1/4 cup of grated Parmesan cheese
- 1/4 teaspoon of dried basil
- 1/4 teaspoon of dried oregano
- Salt and pepper, to taste
- 1 tablespoon of olive oil

Instructions:

1. Preheat the oven to 400°F (200°C). Line a baking sheet with parchment paper.
2. In a small bowl, mix together minced garlic, shredded mozzarella cheese, grated

Parmesan cheese, dried basil, dried oregano, salt, and pepper.

3. Spread the cheese mixture on the slices of bread.

4. Cut the bread into halves or quarters, depending on your desired size.

5. Place the bread slices on the prepared baking sheet.

6. Brush the bread with olive oil.

7. Bake for 10-15 minutes or until the cheese is melted and the bread is golden brown.

8. Serve hot and enjoy!

Nutritional Information (per serving):

- Calories: 315
- Total Fat: 19g
- Saturated Fat: 6g
- Cholesterol: 24mg
- Sodium: 772mg
- Total Carbohydrates: 22g
- Dietary Fiber: 2g
- Sugar: 2g
- Protein: 14g

Benefits of the Diet:

- The recipe contains whole grain bread which is a good source of fiber and can help regulate blood sugar levels.

- The use of cheese in the recipe adds flavor and richness while also providing a source of calcium and protein.

- Olive oil is a healthier fat option compared to other oils, and has a beneficial effect on heart health.

- Garlic is a flavorful addition to the recipe and has numerous health benefits,

including potential antibacterial and antiviral properties.

Microwave Sweet Potato Chips

Preparation Time: 5 minutes

Serving: 2

Ingredients:

- 2 medium-sized sweet potatoes
- 1 tablespoon olive oil
- Salt and pepper to taste

Instructions:

1. Wash and peel the sweet potatoes, then thinly slice them into rounds.

2. In a large bowl, toss the sweet potato slices with olive oil, salt, and pepper.

3. Place the sweet potato slices in a single layer on a large microwave-safe plate.

4. Microwave on high for 4-5 minutes, or until the sweet potatoes are crispy and lightly browned.

5. Serve the sweet potato chips as a snack or side dish.

Nutritional Information (per serving): Calories: 140 Total Fat: 7g Saturated Fat: 1g Cholesterol: 0mg Sodium: 120mg Total Carbohydrates: 20g Dietary Fiber: 3g Sugar: 5g Protein: 2g

Benefit of the diet: Sweet potatoes are a good source of carbohydrates and fiber, which are important for regulating blood sugar levels. They are also rich in vitamins and minerals, including vitamin A, vitamin C, and potassium. Eating sweet potato chips as a snack or side dish can help provide a boost of nutrients and energy for people with diabetes. Additionally, microwaving the sweet potato chips instead of deep-frying them reduces the amount of unhealthy fat and calories, making this a healthier option for people with diabetes.

Vegetable Pizza Squares

Preparation Time: 20 minutes **Serving:** 2

Ingredients:

- 1/2 cup whole wheat flour
- 1/2 teaspoon baking powder
- 1/4 teaspoon salt
- 1 large egg
- 1/4 cup milk
- 1/4 cup tomato sauce
- 1/4 teaspoon dried oregano
- 1/4 teaspoon dried basil
- 1/4 teaspoon garlic powder
- 1/2 cup shredded mozzarella cheese
- 1/4 cup chopped bell peppers
- 1/4 cup chopped mushrooms
- 1/4 cup chopped onions

Instructions:

1. Preheat the oven to 400°F (200°C). Line a baking sheet with parchment paper.

2. In a large bowl, mix together the flour, baking powder, and salt.

3. In a separate bowl, beat the egg and add the milk. Pour the mixture into the dry ingredients and stir until well combined.

4. Stir in the tomato sauce, oregano, basil, garlic powder, cheese, bell peppers, mushrooms, and onions.

5. Pour the mixture into the prepared baking sheet and spread it evenly to make a rectangular shape.

6. Bake for 15-20 minutes or until the edges are golden brown and the cheese is melted.

7. Remove from the oven and let it cool for 5 minutes. Cut into squares and serve.

Nutritional Information (per serving):

- Calories: 220
- Fat: 10 g
- Saturated Fat: 4 g
- Cholesterol: 95 mg
- Sodium: 660 mg
- Carbohydrates: 21 g
- Fiber: 4 g
- Sugar: 6 g
- Protein: 14 g

Benefit of the diet: This recipe is a great option for people with diabetes because it is low in carbohydrates, which helps to control blood sugar levels. The use of whole wheat flour instead of regular flour and the addition of vegetables make it a nutritious and filling meal. The fiber in the vegetables and the protein from the cheese and eggs help to regulate the digestion and keep you feeling full for longer.

Apple-Cheddar Quesadillas Recipe:

Preparation Time: 10 minutes

 Serving: 2

Ingredients:

- 2 whole wheat tortillas
- 1 small Granny Smith apple, cored and thinly sliced
- 1/2 cup shredded cheddar cheese
- 1 tablespoon olive oil

- 1 tablespoon honey mustard sauce (or regular mustard)

Instructions:

1. Preheat a large skillet over medium heat.
2. Place a tortilla on a flat surface and spread half of the cheese evenly over it.
3. Arrange half of the apple slices on top of the cheese.
4. Repeat with the remaining tortilla, cheese, and apple slices.
5. Brush both sides of the tortillas with olive oil.
6. Place one quesadilla in the skillet and cook for 2-3 minutes on each side, or until the cheese is melted and the tortilla is golden brown.
7. Repeat with the second quesadilla.
8. Cut each quesadilla into wedges and serve with honey mustard sauce.

Nutritional Information (per serving):

- Calories: 377
- Fat: 17g
- Saturated Fat: 8g
- Carbohydrates: 41g
- Fiber: 4g
- Sugar: 15g
- Protein: 15g

Benefits of the Diet:

1. Whole wheat tortillas provide fiber to help regulate blood sugar levels.
2. Apples are a low-glycemic fruit that helps prevent spikes in blood sugar levels.
3. Cheddar cheese is a good source of protein, which helps keep you feeling full and satisfied.

4. Olive oil is a healthy source of monounsaturated fats, which can help improve insulin sensitivity.
5. Honey mustard is a low-sugar alternative to traditional high-sugar condiments.

Texas Cheese Dip Recipe:

Preparation Time: 10 minutes

Servings: 2

Ingredients:

- 1 cup shredded cheddar cheese
- 1/2 cup shredded mozzarella cheese
- 1/4 cup diced onion
- 1/4 cup diced green bell pepper
- 2 tablespoons diced jalapeño pepper
- 1/2 cup diced tomato
- 1/4 teaspoon garlic powder
- 1/4 teaspoon chili powder
- Salt and pepper, to taste
- 4 whole-grain tortilla chips, for serving

Instructions:

1. In a microwave-safe bowl, mix together the cheddar cheese, mozzarella cheese, onion, green bell pepper, jalapeño pepper, tomato, garlic powder, chili powder, salt, and pepper.
2. Cover the bowl with a microwave-safe plate and microwave on high for 2 minutes.
3. Remove the plate and stir the cheese mixture.
4. Replace the plate and microwave for another 2 minutes, or until the cheese is melted and bubbly.

5. Serve with whole-grain tortilla chips.

Nutritional Information (per serving):

- Calories: 360
- Fat: 25g
- Saturated Fat: 14g
- Cholesterol: 70mg
- Sodium: 700mg
- Carbohydrates: 15g
- Fiber: 3g
- Sugar: 3g
- Protein: 19g

The benefit of this diabetic-friendly recipe is that it uses whole-grain tortilla chips for dipping, which provides fiber and helps regulate blood sugar levels. Additionally, the use of vegetables such as onions, bell peppers, and jalapeño peppers adds a serving of nutritious veggies to the dish, helping to meet daily fiber and vitamin requirements.

New Delhi Dip Recipe:

Preparation Time: 10 minutes

Serving: 2 people

Ingredients:

- 1 cup of plain Greek yogurt
- 1 tablespoon grated fresh ginger
- 1 small clove garlic, minced
- 1 tablespoon chili powder
- 1 tablespoon cumin
- 1/2 tablespoon coriander
- 1/2 tablespoon garam masala
- 1/4 tablespoon turmeric
- Salt, to taste
- 1/2 lemon, juiced
- 1/4 cup of fresh cilantro, chopped
- 1/2 cucumber, chopped

Instructions:

1. In a medium bowl, mix together the Greek yogurt, grated ginger, minced garlic, chili powder, cumin, coriander, garam masala, turmeric, salt, and lemon juice.
2. Stir in the chopped cilantro.
3. Serve the dip with chopped cucumber for dipping.

Nutritional Information per **Serving:** Calories: 80 Protein: 10g Fat: 3g Carbohydrates: 6g Fiber: 2g

Benefits of the Diet: This New Delhi Dip is a perfect low-carb, high-protein snack option for people with diabetes. The Greek yogurt is a good source of protein, while the spices and herbs used in this recipe provide flavor without adding extra sugar. The cucumber used as a dip is low in carbohydrates and high in fiber, which helps to regulate blood sugar levels. This dip is a great option for those looking for a tasty and nutritious snack that can help control blood

Vegetable Dip Recipe

Preparation Time: 10 minutes

Serving: 2

Ingredients:

- 1 cup Greek yogurt
- 1 clove of garlic, minced
- 2 tablespoons fresh lemon juice
- 2 tablespoons chopped fresh dill
- Salt and pepper, to taste
- Assorted vegetables for dipping (carrots, bell peppers, cucumber, etc.)

Instructions:

1. In a medium bowl, mix together the Greek yogurt, minced garlic, lemon juice, and dill.

2. Season with salt and pepper, to taste.

3. Cover and chill in the refrigerator for at least 30 minutes.

4. Serve with an assortment of vegetables for dipping.

Nutritional Information (per serving):

- Calories: 85
- Total Fat: 5g
- Saturated Fat: 3g
- Cholesterol: 20mg
- Sodium: 210mg
- Total Carbohydrates: 5g
- Dietary Fiber: 2g
- Sugar: 3g
- Protein: 7g

Benefit of the diet: This Vegetable Dip recipe is a great option for people with diabetes as it is low in carbohydrates and high in protein. The use of Greek yogurt instead of sour cream helps to lower the fat content and increase the protein. Vegetables are a great source of fiber and vitamins and are a low-carb option for dipping, making this a healthy snack choice. The addition of garlic, lemon juice, and dill add flavor without adding many extra calories.

Black Bean Salsa

Preparation Time: 10 minutes

Serving: 2

Ingredients:

- 1 can black beans, rinsed and drained
- 1 medium tomato, diced
- 1/2 medium red onion, finely chopped
- 1 medium jalapeno, seeded and finely chopped
- 2 tablespoon chopped fresh cilantro
- 1 tablespoon fresh lime juice
- 1/2 tablespoon ground cumin
- Salt and pepper to taste

Instructions:

1. In a medium bowl, combine all the ingredients, black beans, diced tomato, chopped red onion, jalapeno, cilantro, lime juice, cumin, salt, and pepper.

2. Mix well until all the ingredients are evenly combined.

3. Cover the bowl and refrigerate the salsa for at least 30 minutes to allow the flavors to meld.

4. Serve with your favorite chips, or as a topping for tacos, burritos, or salads.

Nutritional Information (per serving): Calories: 107 Total Fat: 1 g Saturated Fat: 0 g Cholesterol: 0 mg Sodium: 258 mg Total Carbohydrates: 21 g Dietary Fiber: 7 g Sugars: 2 g Protein: 7 g

Benefits of the Diet:

- The black beans in this recipe are an excellent source of fiber, which can help regulate blood sugar levels.

- Tomatoes, red onions, and jalapenos are all low-glycemic index foods that can help regulate blood sugar levels and reduce insulin resistance.

- The fresh cilantro provides a source of antioxidants, which can help protect the body from cellular damage caused by free radicals.

- The lime juice and cumin add a burst of flavor and help keep the salsa low in calories and sodium.

Fruit Leather

Preparation Time: 10 minutes

Serving: 2

Ingredients:

- 2 cups of your favorite fresh or frozen fruit (strawberries, blueberries, raspberries, peaches, etc.)
- 2 tablespoons of honey (optional)
- 1 teaspoon of lemon juice (optional)

Instructions:

1. Preheat your oven to its lowest setting, typically between 150°F and 200°F.
2. If using frozen fruit, let it thaw until soft.
3. Puree the fruit in a blender or food processor.
4. Stir in the honey and lemon juice (if using) until well combined.
5. Pour the mixture onto a silicone mat or parchment paper-lined baking sheet.
6. Spread it evenly, about 1/8 inch thick.
7. Bake for 4 to 6 hours, or until the fruit leather is no longer sticky and can be easily lifted from the mat or parchment paper.
8. Allow to cool completely, then peel away from the mat or parchment paper and cut into strips.

Nutritional Information (per serving):

- Calories: 75
- Total Fat: 0g
- Sodium: 1mg
- Total Carbohydrates: 19g
- Dietary Fiber: 2g
- Sugars: 16g
- Protein: 1g

The **Benefit of the diet:** Fruit leather is a low-calorie, low-fat snack that is high in fiber and antioxidants. This snack is an excellent alternative to processed, high-fat snacks that are often high in added sugars and low in nutrients. Additionally, fruit leather is easy to make and store, making it a great option for those with a busy lifestyle.

Sweet Potato Chips in the Air Fryer Recipe

Preparation Time: 15 minutes

Cooking Time: 15 minutes

Serving: 2

Ingredients:

- 2 medium-sized sweet potatoes, sliced into 1/8 inch rounds
- 1 tablespoon olive oil
- 1 tablespoon salt
- 1 tablespoon black pepper
- 1 tablespoon paprika

Instructions:

1. Preheat the air fryer to 400°F.
2. Slice the sweet potatoes into 1/8 inch rounds.
3. Place the slices in a bowl and add the olive oil, salt, pepper, and paprika. Mix well to ensure that all the slices are coated.
4. Place the sweet potato slices in the air fryer in a single layer, making sure that they are not touching.

5. Cook for 15 minutes or until the chips are crispy and golden brown, flipping the chips over halfway through cooking.

6. Serve immediately and enjoy!

Nutritional Information (per serving): Calories: 200 Protein: 2g Carbohydrates: 36g Fat: 7g

Benefit of the diet:

- Sweet potatoes are a good source of fiber, vitamins, and minerals, making them a great option for people with diabetes.

- Using an air fryer to cook the sweet potato chips is a healthier alternative to traditional deep-frying, as it reduces the amount of oil used.

- This recipe is low in carbohydrates, making it a good option for people with diabetes who are trying to manage their blood sugar levels.

Jicama Appetizer Recipe for Diabetics

Preparation Time: 10 minutes

Serving: 2

Ingredients:

- 1 medium-sized jicama, peeled and cut into thin slices

- 2 tablespoon fresh lime juice

- 1 tablespoon chili powder

- Salt and pepper to taste

- 2 tablespoon chopped fresh cilantro (optional)

Instructions:

1. Preheat the air fryer to 400°F.

2. In a large bowl, mix the jicama slices with the lime juice, chili powder, salt, and pepper.

3. Arrange the jicama slices in a single layer in the air fryer basket.

4. Cook for 10 minutes or until crispy and slightly browned.

5. Serve hot and sprinkle with chopped cilantro if desired.

Nutritional Information (per serving): Calories: 75 Fat: 0.5g Carbohydrates: 17g Protein: 2g Fiber: 7g

The benefit of this diet: Jicama is a low-carb and low-calorie vegetable that is a good source of fiber. This recipe is a tasty and healthy snack option for people with diabetes, as it provides a satisfying crunch without spikes in blood sugar levels. The fiber in jicama also helps regulate digestion and lower cholesterol levels. Additionally, the chili powder and lime juice add flavor and antioxidants to the dish.

Mexican Jicama Snack

Preparation Time: 10 minutes

Serving: 2

Ingredients:

- 1 large jicama, peeled and sliced into sticks

- 1 tablespoon lime juice

- 1 tablespoon chili powder

- Salt, to taste

- 1 tablespoon chopped cilantro (optional)

Instructions:

1. In a bowl, mix together the lime juice, chili powder, and salt.

2. Add in the jicama sticks and toss to coat evenly.

3. Place jicama sticks on a serving platter and sprinkle with cilantro, if desired.

Nutritional Information (per serving):

- Calories: 72
- Carbohydrates: 17 g
- Protein: 1 g
- Fat: 0 g
- Fiber: 6 g

Benefits of the Diet: Jicama is a low-carb vegetable that is high in fiber and low in calories, making it an excellent snack for people with diabetes. The high fiber content helps regulate blood sugar levels and promotes feelings of fullness. The addition of chili powder and lime juice add flavor and antioxidants to this healthy snack.

Pineapple Salsa Recipe

Preparation Time: 15 minutes

Serving: 2

Ingredients:

- 1 cup diced pineapple
- 1/2 red bell pepper, diced
- 1/2 jalapeño pepper, seeded and diced
- 1 small red onion, diced
- 1 tablespoon freshly squeezed lime juice
- 1 tablespoon chopped fresh cilantro
- Salt, to taste

Instructions:

1. In a medium bowl, mix together the diced pineapple, red bell pepper, jalapeño pepper, red onion, lime juice, and cilantro.
2. Season with salt, to taste.
3. Cover and refrigerate for at least 30 minutes to allow the flavors to meld.
4. Serve with chips or as a topping for tacos or grilled meats.

Nutritional Information (per serving):

- Calories: 60
- Total Fat: 0.5g
- Sodium: 3mg
- Total Carbohydrates: 15g
- Dietary Fiber: 2g
- Sugars: 11g
- Protein: 1g

The Benefit of this Diet:

- Low in calories and high in fiber, this salsa is a healthy option for those with diabetes.
- Pineapple is a good source of vitamin C and other antioxidants, which can help support overall health.
- Using fresh ingredients, like jalapeño peppers, red onions, and cilantro, provides a flavorful, healthy alternative to traditional high-fat dips.

Banana Oat Energy Bars

Preparation Time: 20 minutes

Serving: 2

Ingredients:

- 1 ripe banana, mashed
- 1 cup oats
- 1/4 cup almond butter
- 1/4 cup honey
- 1 tablespoon cinnamon
- 1/2 tablespoon vanilla extract
- 1/4 tablespoon salt
- 1/2 cup chopped nuts (optional)
- 1/2 cup dried fruit (optional)

Instructions:

1. Preheat the oven to 350°F. Line a 9x9 inch baking dish with parchment paper.
2. In a medium bowl, mix together the mashed banana, oats, almond butter, honey, cinnamon, vanilla extract, and salt until well combined.
3. Stir in the chopped nuts and dried fruit if desired.
4. Press the mixture evenly into the prepared baking dish.
5. Bake for 15-20 minutes, or until the edges are golden brown.

6. Let the bars cool in the dish for 10 minutes, then remove and let cool completely on a wire rack.

7. Cut into squares and serve.

Nutritional Information (per serving, based on 2 servings): Calories: 400 Fat: 19g Protein: 10g Carbohydrates: 53g Fiber: 6g

Benefits of the Diet:

- The oats and almond butter in this recipe provide slow-digesting carbohydrates to help manage blood sugar levels.

- The use of honey as a sweetener helps keep the sugar content lower compared to traditional recipes that use white sugar.

- The inclusion of nuts and dried fruit adds healthy fats and fiber to the bars, making them a more filling and nutritious snack.

Spicy Lentil Guacamole

Preparation Time: 20 minutes

Serving: 2

Ingredients:

- 1 cup cooked brown lentils
- 1 ripe avocado
- 1 jalapeno pepper, seeded and chopped
- 1 small clove garlic, minced
- 1 small lime, juiced
- Salt, to taste
- 1 small tomato, diced
- 2 tablespoons chopped fresh cilantro

Instructions:

1. In a medium bowl, mash the avocado.

2. Add the cooked lentils, jalapeno, garlic, lime juice, and salt. Mash everything together until well combined.

3. Stir in the diced tomato and cilantro.

4. Serve with whole grain crackers or use as a spread for sandwiches.

Nutritional Information (per serving):

- Calories: 220
- Fat: 11g
- Saturated Fat: 1.5g
- Cholesterol: 0mg
- Sodium: 140mg
- Carbohydrates: 28g
- Fiber: 12g
- Sugar: 2g
- Protein: 10g

The benefit of this diet: This recipe is a great option for people with diabetes as it is low in carbohydrates and high in fiber. Lentils are a good source of protein and fiber, which can help regulate blood sugar levels and keep you feeling full for longer. Avocados are also a healthy source of unsaturated fats, which can help lower cholesterol levels. This dish is a tasty and nutritious way to add more plant-based ingredients to your diet.

Chocolate Cake Batter Hummus Recipe

Preparation Time: 10 minutes

Serving: 2

Ingredients:

- 1 can chickpeas, drained and rinsed
- 1/4 cup unsweetened cocoa powder
- 1/4 cup almond butter

- 2 tablespoon honey
- 1 tablespoon vanilla extract
- 1/4 tablespoon salt
- 2 tablespoon almond milk

Instructions:

1. In a food processor, combine chickpeas, cocoa powder, almond butter, honey, vanilla extract, and salt.
2. Process until smooth, scraping down the sides as needed.
3. Add in the almond milk, and continue processing until well combined.
4. Serve with your favorite dippers, such as fruit, crackers, or veggies.

Nutritional Information (per serving): Calories: 361 Fat: 19g Carbohydrates: 43g Protein: 11g Fiber: 8g

Benefit of the diet: Including hummus in your diet can be beneficial for people with diabetes as it is a good source of protein, fiber, and healthy fats. This chocolate cake batter hummus recipe is lower in sugar compared to traditional dessert hummus recipes, making it a great option for those following a diabetic-friendly diet.

Mango Ceviche Recipe:

Preparation Time: 20 minutes + chilling time Servings: 2

Ingredients:

- 2 ripe mangoes, peeled, pitted and diced
- 1/2 red onion, diced
- 1 jalapeño pepper, seeded and minced
- 1/4 cup fresh lime juice
- 1/4 cup fresh lemon juice
- 2 tablespoons fresh cilantro, chopped
- Salt and pepper to taste

- 2 tablespoon olive oil
- Crackers or vegetables for serving (optional)

Instructions:

1. In a large bowl, mix together the mangoes, red onion, jalapeño pepper, lime juice, lemon juice, and cilantro.
2. Season with salt and pepper to taste.
3. Cover the bowl with plastic wrap and refrigerate for at least 2 hours or overnight.
4. Before serving, remove the ceviche from the refrigerator and drizzle with olive oil.
5. Serve with crackers or vegetables, if desired.

Nutritional Information (per serving):

- Calories: 190
- Fat: 9g
- Saturated Fat: 1g
- Cholesterol: 0mg
- Sodium: 35mg
- Carbohydrates: 28g
- Fiber: 3g
- Sugar: 22g
- Protein: 3g

Benefit of the diet:

- Mango ceviche is a great option for diabetics as it is low in carbohydrates and high in fiber, making it a good choice for stabilizing blood sugar levels.
- The high levels of vitamin C in mangoes help the body absorb iron, which is essential for people with diabetes.

- The jalapeño pepper in the recipe contains capsaicin, a natural substance that may help regulate blood sugar levels.

- The use of lemon and lime juice in the recipe adds flavor while keeping the dish low in sugar.

Spicy Cranberry Salsa

Preparation Time: 15 minutes

Serving: 2

Ingredients:

- 1 cup fresh cranberries

- 1 jalapeño pepper, seeded and finely chopped

- 1/2 red onion, finely chopped

- 1/2 red bell pepper, finely chopped

- 2 tablespoons fresh lime juice

- 1 tablespoon honey

- 1 tablespoon chopped fresh cilantro

- Salt and pepper to taste

Instructions:

1. In a medium bowl, mix together the cranberries, jalapeño, red onion, red bell pepper, lime juice, honey, and cilantro.

2. Season with salt and pepper to taste.

3. Chill the salsa in the refrigerator for at least 30 minutes before serving.

Nutritional Information (per serving): Calories: 92 Fat: 0g Protein: 1g Carbohydrates: 24g Sugar: 15g Fiber: 4g

The benefit of this diet: This recipe is a low-carb and low-fat option for those with diabetes, making it a great choice for managing blood sugar levels. The high fiber content from the cranberries

and other ingredients helps slow down digestion, promoting stable blood sugar levels. The presence of antioxidants, vitamins, and minerals from the ingredients also supports overall health.

Bacon Wrapped New Potatoes Recipe:

Preparation Time: 15 minutes

Cook Time: 25 minutes

Serving: 2

Ingredients:

- 8 new potatoes

- 8 strips of bacon

- Salt, pepper, and paprika to taste

- Fresh parsley, chopped, for garnish (optional)

Instructions:

1. Preheat oven to 400°F. Line a large baking sheet with parchment paper.

2. Rinse the potatoes and cut into halves.

3. Wrap each potato half with a slice of bacon and secure with a toothpick.

4. Season the potatoes with salt, pepper, and paprika.

5. Place the potatoes onto the prepared baking sheet, seam side down.

6. Bake for 25 minutes, or until the bacon is crispy and the potatoes are tender.

7. Remove the toothpicks and sprinkle with chopped parsley (optional).

8. Serve and enjoy!

Nutritional Information (per serving): Calories: 380 Fat: 26 g Saturated Fat: 8 g Carbohydrates: 26 g Fiber: 3 g Sugar: 1 g Protein: 13 g

The **Benefit of the diet:** This dish is high in fiber from the potatoes, and the bacon adds some healthy unsaturated fat. The fiber helps regulate blood sugar levels, which is important for those with diabetes. The dish also provides a good source of protein, which helps keep you feeling full and satisfied. The limited use of seasonings keeps the dish lower in sodium and added sugars, making it a healthy option for those with diabetes.

Asparagus Guacamole Recipe:

Preparation Time: 20 minutes

Serving: 2

Ingredients:

- 1 pound asparagus, trimmed and chopped
- 2 ripe avocados, peeled and pitted
- 2 cloves garlic, minced
- 2 tablespoons lemon juice
- Salt and pepper to taste
- Optional: 1/4 cup chopped cilantro

Instructions:

1. Boil the asparagus in a pot of salted water for 2-3 minutes, or until tender but still crisp. Drain and set aside to cool.

2. In a large bowl, mash the avocados with a fork or potato masher.

3. Add the minced garlic, lemon juice, salt, and pepper to the bowl and mix well.

4. Add the cooled asparagus to the bowl and mix until well combined.

5. Optional: Stir in the chopped cilantro.

6. Serve immediately, or cover and refrigerate until ready to serve.

Nutritional Information (per serving):

- Calories: approximately 256
- Carbohydrates: approximately 21g
- Fat: approximately 22g
- Protein: approximately 4g
- Fiber: approximately 11g

Benefits of the Diet:

- Avocados are a great source of healthy monounsaturated fats and fiber.
- Asparagus is low in carbohydrates and high in fiber, making it a great vegetable for people with diabetes.
- Garlic has been shown to help lower blood sugar levels and improve insulin sensitivity.
- The lemon juice adds a boost of vitamin C and helps to add flavor to the dish without adding many calories or carbohydrates.

This dish is a delicious and nutritious way to enjoy the flavors of the Mediterranean while managing blood sugar levels.

SIDE DISHES

Orange Glazed Carrots Recipe

Preparation Time: 15 minutes

Cooking Time: 20 minutes

Serving: 2 people

Ingredients:

- 1 pound carrots, peeled and sliced into 1/4-inch rounds
- 2 tablespoons olive oil
- 2 tablespoons orange juice
- 1 tablespoon honey

- 1/2 teaspoon salt

- 1/4 teaspoon black pepper

- 1 teaspoon grated orange zest

- 2 tablespoons chopped fresh parsley

Instructions:

1. In a medium saucepan, bring 2 cups of water to a boil. Add the carrots and cook until they are just tender, about 5 minutes. Drain and set aside.

2. In a small saucepan, heat the oil over medium heat. Add the orange juice, honey, salt, and pepper. Stir until the honey has dissolved.

3. Add the orange zest to the saucepan and pour the sauce over the carrots.

4. Preheat the oven to 375°F. Transfer the carrots to a baking dish and roast in the oven until they are golden and glazed, about 15 minutes.

5. Sprinkle the parsley over the carrots and serve.

Nutritional Information (per serving): Calories: 210 Fat: 13g Carbohydrates: 27g Protein: 2g Fiber: 5g Sugar: 17g

The benefit of this diet:

- Carrots are a good source of fiber, which can help regulate blood sugar levels.

- The orange juice and zest add natural sweetness to the dish without adding any added sugars.

- The orange juice also provides vitamin C, which is an antioxidant that can help improve insulin sensitivity.

- Olive oil is a healthy source of monounsaturated fats, which can help improve cholesterol levels and reduce the reduce the risk of heart disease.

Marinated Mushrooms Recipe

Serving: 2

Preparation Time: 20 minutes

Ingredients:

- 8 oz mushrooms, sliced

- 2 tablespoon olive oil

- 2 cloves garlic, minced

- 1 tablespoon balsamic vinegar

- 1 tablespoon lemon juice

- 1 tablespoon dried oregano

- Salt and pepper to taste

Instructions:

1. In a mixing bowl, combine the sliced mushrooms, minced garlic, balsamic vinegar, lemon juice, dried oregano, salt and pepper.

2. In a separate pan, heat the olive oil over medium heat.

3. Add the mushrooms mixture to the pan and sauté for 5-7 minutes or until the mushrooms are tender and fully cooked.

4. Serve hot and enjoy!

Nutritional Information (per serving):

- Calories: 140

- Total Fat: 14g

- Saturated Fat: 2g

- Cholesterol: 0mg

- Sodium: 50mg

- Total Carbohydrates: 5g

- Dietary Fiber: 2g

- Total Sugar: 2g

- Protein: 3g

The **Benefit of the diet:** This dish is a great option for those with diabetes as it is low in carbohydrates and high in fiber. The fiber in mushrooms can help regulate blood sugar levels, while the healthy fats in the olive oil can help keep you feeling full for longer periods of time. Additionally, the balsamic vinegar and lemon juice add a tangy flavor without adding extra sugar to the dish.

Stuffed Potatoes

Preparation Time: 30 minutes

Serving: 2

Ingredients:

- 2 medium potatoes
- 1/4 cup of cooked and diced chicken breast
- 1/4 cup of diced tomatoes
- 1/4 cup of shredded cheese
- 2 tablespoons of diced red onions
- 2 tablespoons of chopped fresh parsley
- Salt and pepper, to taste
- Non-stick cooking spray

Instructions:

1. Preheat the oven to 375°F.
2. Wash and dry the potatoes, then prick them several times with a fork.
3. Place the potatoes on a baking sheet and bake for 25-30 minutes, or until they are tender when pierced with a fork.
4. While the potatoes are cooking, mix the chicken, tomatoes, cheese, red onions, parsley, salt and pepper in a small bowl.
5. Remove the potatoes from the oven and let them cool for 5 minutes.

6. Cut the potatoes in half lengthwise and carefully scoop out the flesh, leaving a 1/4 inch thick shell.
7. Mix the scooped potato flesh with the chicken mixture.
8. Spoon the mixture back into the potato shells and sprinkle with more cheese.
9. Place the stuffed potatoes back on the baking sheet and bake for another 15-20 minutes, or until the cheese is melted and the filling is heated through.
10. Serve immediately.

Nutritional Information (per serving):

- Calories: 330
- Fat: 9 g
- Saturated Fat: 4 g
- Cholesterol: 60 mg
- Sodium: 360 mg
- Carbohydrates: 47 g
- Fiber: 4 g
- Sugar: 4 g
- Protein: 19 g

Benefit of the diet:

- Potatoes are a good source of carbohydrates and provide energy for the body.
- Chicken is a low-fat protein source that helps to repair and build muscle tissue.
- Tomatoes and red onions provide vitamin C, which helps to boost the immune system.
- The cheese provides calcium, which is important for strong bones.
- Parsley is a rich source of antioxidants and helps to protect cells from damage.

Crispy Smashed Balsamic-Parmesan Mushrooms

Preparation Time: 15 minutes

Serving: 2

Ingredients:

- 10 ounces mushrooms, trimmed and wiped clean
- 2 tablespoons olive oil
- 2 tablespoons balsamic vinegar
- 1/4 cup grated parmesan cheese
- Salt and pepper, to taste
- Fresh parsley, chopped, for garnish (optional)

Instructions:

1. Preheat oven to 400°F (200°C). Line a large baking sheet with parchment paper.
2. Place the mushrooms on the prepared baking sheet and gently smash each mushroom using the bottom of a drinking glass or a meat mallet.
3. Drizzle the mushrooms with the olive oil and balsamic vinegar.
4. Sprinkle the parmesan cheese on top and season with salt and pepper.
5. Roast in the oven for 10-15 minutes, or until the mushrooms are crispy and tender.
6. Serve hot, garnished with fresh parsley, if desired.

Nutritional Information (per serving): Calories: 193 Fat: 16.2 g Saturated Fat: 3.6 g Carbohydrates: 7.3 g Fiber: 1.8 g Protein: 8.2 g

Benefit of the diet: This dish is a great option for people with diabetes because it is low in carbohydrates and high in healthy fats and protein. The use of mushrooms as a base provides a good source of fiber and helps to regulate blood sugar levels. The addition of balsamic vinegar and parmesan cheese provides a delicious flavor without adding extra sugar to the dish. Additionally, this recipe is easy to prepare and can be served as a side dish or a snack.

Maple-Roasted Sweet Potatoes

Preparation Time: 15 minutes

Cooking Time: 30 minutes

Serving: 2

Ingredients:

- 2 medium sized sweet potatoes, peeled and cut into 1/2 inch slices
- 2 tablespoons of olive oil
- 2 tablespoons of pure maple syrup
- 1/2 teaspoon of salt
- 1/4 teaspoon of black pepper
- 1/4 teaspoon of cinnamon
- 1/4 teaspoon of nutmeg

Instructions:

1. Preheat the oven to 400°F.
2. In a large mixing bowl, combine the sliced sweet potatoes, olive oil, maple syrup, salt, pepper, cinnamon, and nutmeg. Mix well until the sweet potatoes are evenly coated.
3. Arrange the sweet potatoes in a single layer on a large baking sheet.
4. Bake for 25 to 30 minutes, or until the sweet potatoes are tender and lightly caramelized.
5. Serve hot.

Nutritional Information (per serving):

- Calories: 240
- Total Fat: 9 g
- Saturated Fat: 1 g
- Cholesterol: 0 mg
- Sodium: 330 mg
- Total Carbohydrates: 40 g
- Dietary Fiber: 4 g
- Sugar: 16 g
- Protein: 2 g

Benefit of the diet: Sweet potatoes are a low glycemic index food, which means they can help regulate blood sugar levels for people with diabetes. They are also a good source of fiber, vitamins, and minerals, making them a nutritious and filling food for those with diabetes. The addition of healthy fats from olive oil and the natural sweetness from maple syrup in this recipe provides a balanced meal.

Mock Mashed Potatoes

Preparation Time: 15 minutes

Serving: 2

Ingredients:

- 2 medium cauliflower heads, chopped into small florets
- 2 cloves of garlic, minced
- 1 tablespoon butter or margarine
- 2 tablespoons sour cream
- 2 tablespoons grated Parmesan cheese
- Salt and pepper to taste

Instructions:

1. Steam the chopped cauliflower florets and minced garlic in a steamer basket for about 10 minutes or until tender.

2. Transfer the steamed cauliflower and garlic to a large bowl and mash with a potato masher or fork until smooth.

3. Add the butter or margarine, sour cream, Parmesan cheese, salt, and pepper to the mashed cauliflower and mix until well combined.

4. Serve the mock mashed potatoes immediately and enjoy!

Nutritional Information (per serving):

- Calories: 150
- Fat: 11 g
- Carbohydrates: 11 g
- Protein: 6 g
- Fiber: 4 g

Benefit of the diet: This mock mashed potato recipe is a low-carb alternative to traditional mashed potatoes and is perfect for people with diabetes or those who are trying to maintain a healthy diet. Cauliflower is a nutrient-rich vegetable that is high in fiber and low in carbohydrates, making it a great choice for those with diabetes. The addition of garlic, butter, sour cream, and Parmesan cheese adds flavor and creaminess to the dish, while also helping to keep you feeling full and satisfied.

Roasted Asparagus with Bacon

Preparation Time: 10 minutes

Cooking Time: 20 minutes

Serving: 2 people

Ingredients:

- 1 bunch of asparagus, trimmed

- 4-6 slices of bacon, cut into 1-inch pieces

- 1 tablespoon olive oil

- Salt and pepper, to taste

- Lemon wedges (optional)

Instructions:

1. Preheat the oven to 400°F (200°C). Line a large baking sheet with parchment paper.

2. Place the asparagus and bacon on the prepared baking sheet.

3. Drizzle the olive oil over the asparagus and bacon, then sprinkle with salt and pepper.

4. Toss the asparagus and bacon until evenly coated with oil and seasoning.

5. Roast in the oven for 20 minutes or until the asparagus is tender and the bacon is crispy.

6. Serve hot, garnished with lemon wedges if desired.

Nutritional Information (per serving):

- Calories: 214

- Total Fat: 17g

- Saturated Fat: 5g

- Cholesterol: 20mg

- Sodium: 547mg

- Total Carbohydrates: 10g

- Dietary Fiber: 4g

- Protein: 9g

The **Benefit of the diet:** This dish provides a good source of fiber and protein, which are important components of a healthy diabetic diet. Asparagus is also low in carbohydrates and high in antioxidants, making it a good choice for people with diabetes. The addition of bacon adds flavor and healthy fats to the dish, while the use of olive oil instead of butter helps to keep the saturated fat content low. This dish can be enjoyed as a side or a main dish, and can easily be adjusted to suit children tastes and dietary needs.

Fresh Peas with Mint Recipe

Preparation Time: 10 minutes

Serving: 2

Ingredients:

- 1 cup fresh green peas, shelled

- 2 tablespoons fresh mint leaves, chopped

- 1 tablespoon olive oil

- 1/4 teaspoon salt

- 1/4 teaspoon black pepper

Instructions:

1. Rinse and shell the fresh green peas.

2. In a large skillet, heat the olive oil over medium heat.

3. Add the shelled green peas and cook for 2-3 minutes, or until they are bright green and just tender.

4. Remove the skillet from heat and stir in the chopped mint leaves, salt, and black pepper.

5. Serve immediately, while still warm.

Nutritional Information (per serving): Calories: 116 Fat: 9g Protein: 4g Carbohydrates: 9g Fiber: 3g

The benefit of this diet:

- Fresh green peas are a good source of fiber, protein, vitamins, and minerals, making them an excellent choice for a diabetic diet.

- This recipe also contains fresh mint leaves, which have been shown to have a beneficial effect on blood sugar levels, as well as being a good source of antioxidants.

- The use of olive oil in this recipe provides healthy monounsaturated fats, which can help to lower cholesterol levels and reduce the risk of heart disease.

Roasted Carrots and Parsnips Recipe

Preparation Time: 15 minutes

Cook time: 25 minutes

Servings: 2

Ingredients:

- 2 medium-sized carrots, peeled and cut into thin rounds
- 2 medium-sized parsnips, peeled and cut into thin rounds
- 1 tablespoon olive oil
- Salt and pepper, to taste
- 1 tablespoon. dried thyme
- 1 tablespoon. dried rosemary
- 1 tablespoon. dried basil

Instructions:

1. Preheat the oven to 400°F. Line a baking sheet with parchment paper.
2. In a large bowl, mix together the carrots and parsnips with the olive oil, salt, pepper, thyme, rosemary, and basil.
3. Spread the mixture out evenly on the prepared baking sheet.
4. Roast for 25 minutes or until the carrots and parsnips are tender and slightly golden.
5. Serve hot as a side dish.

Nutritional information per **Serving:** Calories: 150 Fat: 7g Carbohydrates: 22g Protein: 2g Fiber: 5g

Benefits of the Diet:

- Carrots and parsnips are rich in vitamins and minerals, including vitamin C, potassium, and folate.
- They are also low in calories and high in fiber, making them an ideal food for people with diabetes who need to watch their calorie and carbohydrate intake.
- Roasting vegetables helps to bring out their natural sweetness, and the addition of healthy fats from olive oil can help to improve their absorption of fat-soluble vitamins.
- This recipe is also a great source of antioxidants and anti-inflammatory compounds that can help to improve overall health and reduce the risk of chronic diseases.

Baked Beans from Scratch

Preparation Time: 15 minutes

Cooking Time: 2 hours

Servings: 2

Ingredients:

- 1 cup navy beans, rinsed and drained
- 2 garlic cloves, minced
- 1 small onion, diced
- 1 tablespoon olive oil
- 1 teaspoon dried thyme
- 1 teaspoon smoked paprika
- 1/2 teaspoon chili powder
- 1/2 teaspoon salt

- 1/4 teaspoon black pepper
- 1 can (14.5 oz) diced tomatoes
- 1/2 cup water
- 2 tablespoons molasses
- 1 tablespoon apple cider vinegar
- 1 tablespoon Worcestershire sauce

Instructions:

1. Preheat oven to 325°F (165°C).

2. In a medium saucepan, cover navy beans with water and bring to a boil over high heat. Reduce heat and simmer for 2-3 minutes. Remove from heat and let cool.

3. In a large skillet, heat olive oil over medium heat. Add onion and garlic, and cook until softened, about 5 minutes.

4. Add thyme, paprika, chili powder, salt, and pepper to the skillet, and cook for another minute.

5. Stir in diced tomatoes, water, molasses, apple cider vinegar, and Worcestershire sauce.

6. Transfer the mixture to an oven-safe baking dish. Add navy beans to the baking dish and stir to combine.

7. Cover the baking dish with foil and bake for 1 hour. Remove foil and bake for another hour.

8. Serve warm.

Nutritional Information per **Serving:** Calories: 539 Fat: 8 g Saturated Fat: 1 g Cholesterol: 0 mg Sodium: 863 mg Carbohydrates: 98 g Fiber: 25 g Protein: 26 g

Benefits of the Diet:

- Baked beans are a good source of fiber, which is essential for managing blood sugar levels.

- Navy beans are rich in antioxidants and anti-inflammatory compounds, which help to lower the risk of heart disease and type 2 diabetes.

- This dish provides a good source of protein, which can help to regulate blood sugar levels and reduce the risk of diabetic complications.

Baked Beans from Scratch Recipe

Preparation Time: 15 minutes

Cook Time: 2 hours

Serving Size: 2

Ingredients:

- 1 can (15 ounces) navy beans, drained and rinsed
- 1/2 small onion, diced
- 2 cloves garlic, minced
- 1 tablespoon olive oil
- 1/2 cup tomato sauce
- 1 tablespoon molasses
- 2 teaspoons Dijon mustard
- 1 teaspoon dried thyme
- 1/2 teaspoon paprika
- Salt and pepper, to taste
- 1/4 cup water
- 2 slices cooked and crumbled bacon (optional)

Instructions:

1. Preheat oven to 325°F.

2. In a medium saucepan, heat olive oil over medium heat. Add onion and garlic, cook until onion is soft and translucent.

3. Add the tomato sauce, molasses, Dijon mustard, thyme, paprika, salt, and pepper to the pan. Stir to combine.

4. Add the navy beans and water, stir to combine.

5. Pour the mixture into a 9-inch baking dish.

6. Cover the dish with aluminum foil and bake for 1 1/2 hours.

7. Remove the foil and bake for an additional 30 minutes.

8. Sprinkle the crumbled bacon over the top of the beans (optional).

Nutritional Information (per serving): Calories: 244 Total Fat: 7 g Saturated Fat: 2 g Cholesterol: 11 mg Sodium: 726 mg Total Carbohydrates: 37 g Dietary Fiber: 8 g Sugars: 11 g Protein: 11 g

Benefits of the Diet: This recipe is ideal for childrens with diabetes as it contains a good balance of carbohydrates, fiber, and protein, which helps regulate blood sugar levels. The navy beans are a great source of fiber and protein, which makes this dish filling and helps control hunger. Additionally, the spices used in this recipe contain antioxidants that have been shown to help regulate blood sugar levels. Overall, this dish is a great option for those looking to control their blood sugar levels while enjoying a delicious and satisfying meal.

Easy Southern Fried Green Tomatoes Recipe

Preparation Time: 20 minutes

Cook Time: 10 minutes

Serving: 2

Ingredients:

- 2 large green tomatoes, sliced

- 1/4 cup almond flour

- 1/4 cup cornmeal

- 1/2 tablespoon salt

- 1/2 tablespoon black pepper

- 1/4 tablespoon paprika

- 1 egg, beaten

- 1 tablespoon olive oil

Instructions:

1. Preheat your oven to 200°F (95°C).

2. In a shallow bowl, mix together the almond flour, cornmeal, salt, pepper, and paprika.

3. In another bowl, beat the egg.

4. Dip each tomato slice into the beaten egg, then coat with the flour mixture.

5. In a large pan, heat the olive oil over medium heat.

6. Cook the tomato slices for 2-3 minutes on each side, or until golden brown.

7. Transfer the cooked tomatoes to a baking sheet and keep them warm in the oven while you cook the rest.

8. Serve hot with your favorite dipping sauce.

Nutritional Information (per serving):

- Calories: 220

- Fat: 16g

- Saturated Fat: 2g

- Cholesterol: 93mg

- Sodium: 474mg

- Carbohydrates: 14g

- Fiber: 3g

- Sugar: 5g

- Protein: 8g

The **Benefit of the diet:**

- Green tomatoes are a low-carb, low-sugar food, making them a great option for people with diabetes.

- The almond flour and cornmeal used in this recipe are alternative flour options to traditional wheat flour, which can be high in carbohydrates.

- Olive oil is a heart-healthy fat that can help regulate blood

Squash and Green Bean Saute Side Dish Recipe

Preparation Time: 10 minutes

Cook time: 10 minutes

Serving size: 2

Ingredients:

- 1 medium yellow squash, sliced

- 1 medium zucchini, sliced

- 1 cup green beans, trimmed

- 1 tablespoon olive oil

- Salt and pepper, to taste

- 2 garlic cloves, minced

- 1 tablespoon lemon juice

Instructions:

1. Heat the olive oil in a large pan over medium heat.

2. Add the sliced squash and zucchini to the pan and season with salt and pepper.

3. Cook for 5-7 minutes until the vegetables start to soften.

4. Add the green beans to the pan and continue cooking for another 2-3 minutes.

5. Add the minced garlic and lemon juice to the pan and cook for an additional 1-2 minutes.

6. Serve hot as a side dish.

Nutritional Information (per serving): Calories: 129 Fat: 9 g Carbohydrates: 13 g Protein: 4 g Fiber: 4 g

Benefit of the diet: This recipe is a great option for people with diabetes as it contains a balanced ratio of carbohydrates, fiber, and healthy fats. Squash and green beans are excellent sources of fiber, which helps regulate blood sugar levels. Additionally, the use of olive oil and lemon juice provides a healthy source of fat and added flavor without the need for high-calorie condiments.

Caribbean Slaw Recipe

Preparation Time: 15 minutes

Serving: 2

Ingredients:

- 1 medium-sized green cabbage, shredded

- 1 medium-sized red onion, thinly sliced

- 1 red bell pepper, thinly sliced

- 1 large carrot, grated

- 1 large mango, peeled and diced

- 2 tablespoons fresh lime juice

- 2 tablespoons extra-virgin olive oil

- 1 teaspoon honey

- 1 teaspoon ground cumin

- Salt and pepper, to taste

Instructions:

1. In a large mixing bowl, combine the shredded cabbage, sliced onion, sliced red

bell pepper, grated carrot, and diced mango.

2. In a small mixing bowl, whisk together the lime juice, olive oil, honey, ground cumin, salt, and pepper.

3. Pour the dressing over the slaw ingredients in the large mixing bowl and toss to combine.

4. Serve immediately or refrigerate for at least 30 minutes to allow the flavors to develop.

Nutritional Information per **Serving:**

- Calories: 199
- Total Fat: 14g
- Saturated Fat: 2g
- Cholesterol: 0mg
- Sodium: 49mg
- Total Carbohydrates: 19g
- Dietary Fiber: 5g
- Sugars: 12g
- Protein: 3g

Benefits of the Diet:

- This slaw is a great source of fiber, vitamins, and minerals. The fiber in the cabbage and carrots helps regulate blood sugar levels, while the mango provides a natural source of sugar.

- The olive oil used in the dressing provides monounsaturated fats, which can help improve heart health and lower cholesterol levels.

- The lime juice and cumin in the dressing add flavor and anti-inflammatory properties to the dish.

Baked Potato Recipe

Preparation Time: 1 hour

Servings: 2

Ingredients:

- 2 medium-sized russet potatoes
- Salt and pepper to taste
- 1 tablespoon olive oil

Instructions:

1. Preheat the oven to 400°F (200°C).

2. Wash the potatoes thoroughly and pat them dry.

3. Prick the potatoes several times with a fork to prevent them from bursting.

4. Rub the potatoes with olive oil and season with salt and pepper.

5. Place the potatoes on a baking sheet and bake for 45-60 minutes, or until the skin is crispy and the inside is soft and fluffy.

6. Serve the baked potatoes with your favorite toppings such as sour cream, chives, cheese, or butter.

Nutritional Information per **Serving:**

- Calories: 239
- Total Fat: 7 g
- Saturated Fat: 1 g
- Cholesterol: 0 mg
- Sodium: 21 mg
- Total Carbohydrates: 44 g
- Dietary Fiber: 4 g
- Sugar: 2 g
- Protein: 5 g

The benefit of this diet:

- Baked potatoes are a great source of complex carbohydrates, which provide a slow and steady release of energy.

- They are also low in fat and high in fiber, making them a great option for people with diabetes who are looking to regulate their blood sugar levels.

- The addition of olive oil to the potatoes provides healthy monounsaturated fats, which can help lower cholesterol levels and reduce the risk of heart disease.

SALADS

Broccoli Salad Recipe

Preparation Time: 20 minutes

Servings: 2

Ingredients:

- 2 heads of broccoli florets, chopped
- 1/2 cup raisins
- 1/2 cup diced red onion
- 1/2 cup diced carrots
- 1/2 cup chopped walnuts
- 1/2 cup plain non-fat Greek yogurt
- 2 tablespoons apple cider vinegar
- 2 tablespoons honey
- 1 tablespoon Dijon mustard
- salt and pepper, to taste

Instructions:

1. In a large bowl, mix together the chopped broccoli, raisins, red onion, carrots, and chopped walnuts.

2. In a separate bowl, whisk together the Greek yogurt, apple cider vinegar, honey, Dijon mustard, salt, and pepper until well combined.

3. Pour the dressing over the broccoli mixture and toss until evenly coated.

4. Cover the bowl with plastic wrap and refrigerate for at least 30 minutes to allow the flavors to develop.

5. Serve the broccoli salad chilled and enjoy!

Nutritional Information (per serving): Calories: 300 Total Fat: 17g Saturated Fat: 2g Cholesterol: 5mg Sodium: 190mg Total Carbohydrates: 34g Dietary Fiber: 7g Sugars: 21g Protein: 12g

The benefits of this diet:

- Rich in fiber: The broccoli in this salad provides a good source of fiber, which can help regulate digestion and keep you feeling full for longer.

- Low in calories: With only 300 calories per serving, this salad is a great option for those watching their calorie intake.

- Contains antioxidants: Broccoli is a good source of antioxidants, which can help protect your cells from damage and promote overall health.

- Good source of vitamins and minerals: The carrots, red onion, and raisins in this salad provide a variety of vitamins and minerals, including Vitamin A, Vitamin C, and potassium.

- Promotes heart health: The walnuts in this salad contain monounsaturated and polyunsaturated fats, which can help lower cholesterol levels and promote heart health.

Caprese Salad Recipe

Preparation Time: 10 minutes

Servings: 2

Ingredients:

- 2 medium ripe tomatoes, sliced
- 8 ounces fresh mozzarella cheese, sliced
- 1/4 cup fresh basil leaves
- 2 tablespoons olive oil
- 1 tablespoon balsamic vinegar
- salt and pepper, to taste

Instructions:

1. Arrange the sliced tomatoes and mozzarella cheese on a large serving plate.
2. Scatter the fresh basil leaves on top of the cheese and tomatoes.
3. In a small bowl, whisk together the olive oil and balsamic vinegar.
4. Drizzle the dressing over the salad, and season with salt and pepper to taste.
5. Serve immediately and enjoy!

Nutritional Information (per serving): Calories: 365 Total Fat: 28g Saturated Fat: 12g Cholesterol: 55mg Sodium: 500mg Total Carbohydrates: 6g Dietary Fiber: 1g Sugars: 4g Protein: 22g

The benefits of this diet:

- Low in carbohydrates: With only 6 grams of carbohydrates per serving, this salad is a great option for those following a low-carbohydrate diet.
- Good source of protein: The mozzarella cheese in this salad provides a good source of protein, which can help keep you feeling full and satisfied.
- Rich in healthy fats: The olive oil in this salad is rich in healthy monounsaturated fats, which can help lower cholesterol levels and promote heart health.

- Contains antioxidants: The balsamic vinegar in this salad is a good source of antioxidants, which can help protect your cells from damage and promote overall health.
- Promotes gut health: The basil in this salad is a good source of prebiotics, which can help promote the growth of beneficial bacteria in your gut.

Apple and Celery Salad Recipe

Preparation Time: 10 minutes

Servings: 2

Ingredients:

- 2 medium apples, chopped
- 4 stalks of celery, chopped
- 1/4 cup chopped walnuts
- 2 tablespoons lemon juice
- 2 tablespoons honey
- 1/4 cup plain non-fat Greek yogurt
- salt and pepper, to taste

Instructions:

1. In a large bowl, mix together the chopped apples and celery.
2. Add the chopped walnuts to the bowl and mix well.
3. In a small bowl, whisk together the lemon juice, honey, Greek yogurt, salt, and pepper until well combined.
4. Pour the dressing over the apple and celery mixture and toss until evenly coated.
5. Cover the bowl with plastic wrap and refrigerate for at least 30 minutes to allow the flavors to develop.

6. Serve the apple and celery salad chilled and enjoy!

Nutritional Information (per serving): Calories: 210 Total Fat: 9g Saturated Fat: 1g Cholesterol: 5mg Sodium: 95mg Total Carbohydrates: 31g Dietary Fiber: 5g Sugars: 22g Protein: 5g

The benefits of this diet:

- Low in calories: With only 210 calories per serving, this salad is a great option for those watching their calorie intake.

- Rich in fiber: The apples and celery in this salad provide a good source of fiber, which can help regulate digestion and keep you feeling full for longer.

- Good source of vitamins and minerals: Apples and celery are both good sources of a variety of vitamins and minerals, including Vitamin C, potassium, and folate.

- Promotes heart health: The walnuts in this salad contain monounsaturated and polyunsaturated fats, which can help lower cholesterol levels and promote heart health.

- Supports healthy skin: The Vitamin C in the apples and celery can help promote healthy skin by fighting against damage from free radicals.

Watermelon Fruit Salad with Lime-Mint Dressing Recipe

Preparation Time: 10 minutes

Servings: 2

Ingredients:

- 4 cups diced watermelon

- 1 cup diced cantaloupe

- 1 cup diced honeydew melon

- 2 tablespoons freshly squeezed lime juice

- 2 tablespoons honey

- 1/4 cup fresh mint leaves, chopped

- salt and pepper, to taste

Instructions:

1. In a large bowl, mix together the diced watermelon, cantaloupe, and honeydew melon.

2. In a small bowl, whisk together the lime juice, honey, chopped mint leaves, salt, and pepper until well combined.

3. Pour the dressing over the fruit mixture and toss until evenly coated.

4. Cover the bowl with plastic wrap and refrigerate for at least 30 minutes to allow the flavors to develop.

5. Serve the watermelon fruit salad chilled and enjoy!

Nutritional Information (per serving): Calories: 150 Total Fat: 0.5g Saturated Fat: 0g Cholesterol: 0mg Sodium: 10mg Total Carbohydrates: 39g Dietary Fiber: 1g Sugars: 34g Protein: 2g

The benefits of this diet:

- Low in calories: With only 150 calories per serving, this salad is a great option for those watching their calorie intake.

- Hydrating: The watermelon in this salad is made up of over 90% water, making it a great way to stay hydrated and replenish fluids lost through sweating.

- Good source of vitamins and minerals: Melons are good sources of vitamins and minerals, including Vitamin C, potassium, and folate.

- Supports healthy skin: The Vitamin C in the melons can help promote healthy skin by fighting against damage from free radicals.

- Supports eye health: The Vitamin A in the melons can help promote eye health and prevent age-related vision issues.

Cherry Cola Jello Salad Recipe

Preparation Time: 10 minutes (plus 4 hours chilling time)

Servings: 2

Ingredients:

- 1 package (85g) of cherry-flavored Jello
- 1 cup boiling water
- 1/2 cup cola
- 1/2 cup cold water
- 1 cup chopped fresh cherries
- 1/4 cup chopped walnuts

Instructions:

1. In a large bowl, combine the cherry Jello and boiling water. Stir until the Jello is fully dissolved.
2. Stir in the cola and cold water until well combined.
3. Pour the Jello mixture into a 9x9 inch square dish or a similar-sized container.
4. Cover the dish with plastic wrap and refrigerate for at least 4 hours or until the Jello is fully set.
5. Once the Jello is set, cut it into squares or use a cookie cutter to cut into desired shapes.
6. Top each Jello piece with chopped cherries and chopped walnuts.
7. Serve chilled and enjoy!

Nutritional Information (per serving): Calories: 140 Total Fat: 6g Saturated Fat: 1g Cholesterol: 0mg Sodium: 85mg Total Carbohydrates: 22g Dietary Fiber: 0g Sugars: 18g Protein: 2g

The benefits of this diet:

- Low in calories: With only 140 calories per serving, this salad is a great option for those watching their calorie intake.
- Good source of vitamins and minerals: Cherries are a good source of vitamins and minerals, including Vitamin C, potassium, and folate.
- Supports heart health: The walnuts in this salad contain monounsaturated and polyunsaturated fats, which can help lower cholesterol levels and promote heart health.
- Supports healthy skin: The Vitamin C in the cherries can help promote healthy skin by fighting against damage from free radicals.

Spinach Salad Recipe

Preparation Time: 10 minutes

Servings: 2

Ingredients:

- 4 cups fresh spinach leaves, washed and dried
- 1/2 cup cherry tomatoes, halved
- 1/4 cup chopped red onion
- 2 tablespoons balsamic vinegar
- 2 tablespoons olive oil
- 1 teaspoon Dijon mustard
- salt and pepper, to taste

Instructions:

1. In a large bowl, mix together the spinach leaves, cherry tomatoes, and chopped red onion.

2. In a small bowl, whisk together the balsamic vinegar, olive oil, Dijon mustard, salt, and pepper until well combined.

3. Pour the dressing over the spinach mixture and toss until evenly coated.

4. Cover the bowl with plastic wrap and refrigerate for at least 30 minutes to allow the flavors to develop.

5. Serve the spinach salad chilled and enjoy!

Nutritional Information (per serving): Calories: 160 Total Fat: 14g Saturated Fat: 2g Cholesterol: 0mg Sodium: 180mg Total Carbohydrates: 8g Dietary Fiber: 2g Sugars: 4g Protein: 3g

The benefits of this diet:

- Low in calories: With only 160 calories per serving, this salad is a great option for those watching their calorie intake.

- Good source of vitamins and minerals: Spinach is a good source of vitamins and minerals, including Vitamin A, Vitamin C, potassium, and folate.

- Supports heart health: The olive oil in this salad is a good source of monounsaturated fats, which can help lower cholesterol levels and promote heart health.

- Supports eye health: The Vitamin A in the spinach can help promote eye health and prevent age-related vision issues.

- Supports healthy skin: The Vitamin C in the spinach can help promote healthy skin by fighting against damage from free radicals.

Pear Salad Recipe

Preparation Time: 10 minutes

Servings: 2

Ingredients:

- 2 ripe pears, cored and diced

- 1 cup baby spinach leaves, washed and dried

- 1/4 cup crumbled blue cheese

- 2 tablespoons balsamic vinegar

- 1 tablespoon olive oil

- salt and pepper, to taste

Instructions:

1. In a large bowl, mix together the diced pears, baby spinach leaves, and crumbled blue cheese.

2. In a small bowl, whisk together the balsamic vinegar, olive oil, salt, and pepper until well combined.

3. Pour the dressing over the pear mixture and toss until evenly coated.

4. Cover the bowl with plastic wrap and refrigerate for at least 30 minutes to allow the flavors to develop.

5. Serve the pear salad chilled and enjoy!

Nutritional Information (per serving): Calories: 200 Total Fat: 14g Saturated Fat: 5g Cholesterol: 20mg Sodium: 220mg Total Carbohydrates: 16g Dietary Fiber: 4g Sugars: 10g Protein: 5g

The benefits of this diet:

- Good source of vitamins and minerals: Pears are a good source of vitamins and minerals, including Vitamin C, potassium, and fiber.

- Supports heart health: The olive oil in this salad is a good source of monounsaturated fats, which can help lower cholesterol levels and promote heart health.

- Supports digestive health: The fiber in the pears can help support digestive health and prevent constipation.

- Supports healthy skin: The Vitamin C in the pears can help promote healthy skin by fighting against damage from free radicals.

Waldorf Salad Recipe

Preparation Time: 15 minutes

Servings: 2

Ingredients:

- 2 medium apples, cored and diced
- 1/2 cup diced celery
- 1/4 cup dried cranberries
- 1/4 cup walnuts, chopped
- 2 tablespoons mayonnaise
- 1 tablespoon lemon juice
- salt and pepper, to taste

Instructions:

1. In a large bowl, mix together the diced apples, diced celery, dried cranberries, and chopped walnuts.

2. In a small bowl, whisk together the mayonnaise, lemon juice, salt, and pepper until well combined.

3. Pour the dressing over the apple mixture and toss until evenly coated.

4. Cover the bowl with plastic wrap and refrigerate for at least 30 minutes to allow the flavors to develop.

5. Serve the Waldorf salad chilled and enjoy!

Nutritional Information (per serving): Calories: 250 Total Fat: 18g Saturated Fat: 2g Cholesterol: 10mg Sodium: 140mg Total Carbohydrates: 24g Dietary Fiber: 4g Sugars: 16g Protein: 3g

The benefits of this diet:

- Good source of vitamins and minerals: Apples are a good source of vitamins and minerals, including Vitamin C, potassium, and fiber.

- Supports heart health: The walnuts in this salad are a good source of polyunsaturated fats, which can help lower cholesterol levels and promote heart health.

- Supports healthy skin: The Vitamin C in the apples can help promote healthy skin by fighting against damage from free radicals.

- Supports weight management: The fiber in the apples can help support weight management by promoting feelings of fullness and reducing overall calorie intake.

Tropical Shrimp Salad Recipe

Preparation Time: 20 minutes

Servings: 2

Ingredients:

- 1 lb cooked and peeled shrimp
- 1 cup diced pineapple
- 1 cup diced mango
- 1/2 cup diced red bell pepper
- 2 tablespoons lime juice
- 1 tablespoon olive oil
- 1 teaspoon honey
- salt and pepper, to taste

Instructions:

1. In a large bowl, mix together the cooked and peeled shrimp, diced pineapple, diced mango, and diced red bell pepper.

2. In a small bowl, whisk together the lime juice, olive oil, honey, salt, and pepper until well combined.

3. Pour the dressing over the shrimp mixture and toss until evenly coated.

4. Cover the bowl with plastic wrap and refrigerate for at least 30 minutes to allow the flavors to develop.

5. Serve the tropical shrimp salad chilled and enjoy!

Nutritional Information (per serving): Calories: 280 Total Fat: 9g Saturated Fat: 1.5g Cholesterol: 215mg Sodium: 450mg Total Carbohydrates: 26g Dietary Fiber: 3g Sugars: 21g Protein: 24g

The benefits of this diet:

- Good source of vitamins and minerals: Pineapple and mango are good sources of vitamins and minerals, including Vitamin C, potassium, and fiber.

- Supports heart health: The olive oil in this salad is a good source of monounsaturated fats, which can help lower cholesterol levels and promote heart health.

- Supports healthy skin: The Vitamin C in the pineapple and mango can help promote healthy skin by fighting against damage from free radicals.

- Supports weight management: The fiber in the pineapple and mango can help support weight management by promoting feelings of fullness and reducing overall calorie intake.

Watermelon Strawberry Tomatillo Salad Recipe

Preparation Time: 10 minutes Servings: 2

Ingredients:

- 2 cups diced watermelon

- 1 cup diced strawberries

- 1/2 cup diced tomatillos

- 2 tablespoons lime juice

- 1 tablespoon honey

- salt and pepper, to taste

Instructions:

1. In a large bowl, mix together the diced watermelon, diced strawberries, and diced tomatillos.

2. In a small bowl, whisk together the lime juice, honey, salt, and pepper until well combined.

3. Pour the dressing over the fruit mixture and toss until evenly coated.

4. Cover the bowl with plastic wrap and refrigerate for at least 30 minutes to allow the flavors to develop.

5. Serve the watermelon strawberry tomatillo salad chilled and enjoy!

Nutritional Information (per serving): Calories: 150 Total Fat: 0g Saturated Fat: 0g Cholesterol: 0mg Sodium: 5mg Total Carbohydrates: 39g Dietary Fiber: 2g Sugars: 33g Protein: 2g

The benefits of this diet:

- Good source of vitamins and minerals: Watermelon, strawberries, and tomatillos are good sources of vitamins and minerals, including Vitamin C, potassium, and fiber.

- Supports hydration: The high water content in watermelon can help support hydration, especially during hot weather.

- Supports healthy skin: The Vitamin C in the watermelon, strawberries, and tomatillos can help promote healthy skin by fighting against damage from free radicals.

- Supports weight management: The fiber in the watermelon, strawberries, and tomatillos can help support weight management by promoting feelings of fullness and reducing overall calorie intake.

Chinese Chicken Salad with Sesame Dressing Recipe

Preparation Time: 20 minutes

Servings: 2

Ingredients:

- 2 cups shredded cooked chicken
- 2 cups mixed greens
- 1 cup shredded carrots
- 1/2 cup sliced red bell pepper
- 2 tablespoons sesame oil
- 2 tablespoons rice vinegar
- 1 tablespoon soy sauce
- 1 teaspoon honey
- 1 teaspoon sesame seeds
- salt and pepper, to taste

Instructions:

1. In a large bowl, mix together the shredded cooked chicken, mixed greens, shredded carrots, and sliced red bell pepper.

2. In a small bowl, whisk together the sesame oil, rice vinegar, soy sauce, honey, salt, and pepper until well combined.

3. Pour the dressing over the chicken mixture and toss until evenly coated.

4. Sprinkle the sesame seeds over the top and toss again.

5. Cover the bowl with plastic wrap and refrigerate for at least 30 minutes to allow the flavors to develop.

6. Serve the Chinese chicken salad with sesame dressing chilled and enjoy!

Nutritional Information (per serving): Calories: 420 Total Fat: 22g Saturated Fat: 3g Cholesterol: 95mg Sodium: 1180mg Total Carbohydrates: 12g Dietary Fiber: 2g Sugars: 8g Protein: 37g

The benefits of this diet:

- Good source of protein: The cooked chicken in this salad provides a good source of lean protein, which can help support muscle mass and repair.

- Supports healthy skin: The Vitamin A in the carrots and red bell pepper can help promote healthy skin.

- Supports weight management: The fiber in the mixed greens, carrots, and red bell pepper can help support weight management by promoting feelings of fullness and reducing overall calorie intake.

- Supports heart health: The sesame oil in the dressing is a good source of monounsaturated fats, which can help lower cholesterol levels and promote heart health.

Mandarin Orange Salad Recipe

Preparation Time: 10 minutes

Servings: 2

Ingredients:

- 2 cups mixed greens
- 1 can mandarin oranges, drained

- 1/4 cup chopped walnuts
- 2 tablespoons olive oil
- 2 tablespoons balsamic vinegar
- 1 tablespoon honey
- salt and pepper, to taste

Instructions:

1. In a large bowl, mix together the mixed greens, mandarin oranges, and chopped walnuts.

2. In a small bowl, whisk together the olive oil, balsamic vinegar, honey, salt, and pepper until well combined.

3. Pour the dressing over the mixed greens mixture and toss until evenly coated.

4. Cover the bowl with plastic wrap and refrigerate for at least 30 minutes to allow the flavors to develop.

5. Serve the mandarin orange salad chilled and enjoy!

Nutritional Information (per serving): Calories: 270 Total Fat: 22g Saturated Fat: 2g Cholesterol: 0mg Sodium: 70mg Total Carbohydrates: 19g Dietary Fiber: 2g Sugars: 15g Protein: 3g

The benefits of this diet:

- Good source of vitamin C: The mandarin oranges in this salad are a good source of vitamin C, which can help support the immune system and promote healthy skin.

- Supports healthy fats: The olive oil in the dressing is a good source of monounsaturated fats, which can help lower cholesterol levels and promote heart health.

- Supports weight management: The fiber in the mixed greens and mandarin oranges can help support weight management by promoting feelings of fullness and reducing overall calorie intake.

- Supports blood sugar control: The honey in the dressing provides a natural source of sweetness, which can help support blood sugar control.

Triple Berry Spinach Salad Recipe

Preparation Time: 10 minutes

Servings: 2

Ingredients:

- 2 cups fresh spinach leaves
- 1/2 cup fresh strawberries, sliced
- 1/2 cup fresh blueberries
- 1/2 cup fresh raspberries
- 1/4 cup chopped pecans
- 2 tablespoons olive oil
- 2 tablespoons balsamic vinegar
- 1 tablespoon honey
- salt and pepper, to taste

Instructions:

1. In a large bowl, mix together the spinach leaves, strawberries, blueberries, raspberries, and chopped pecans.

2. In a small bowl, whisk together the olive oil, balsamic vinegar, honey, salt, and pepper until well combined.

3. Pour the dressing over the mixed greens mixture and toss until evenly coated.

4. Cover the bowl with plastic wrap and refrigerate for at least 30 minutes to allow the flavors to develop.

5. Serve the triple berry spinach salad chilled and enjoy!

Nutritional Information (per serving): Calories: 270 Total Fat: 22g Saturated Fat: 2g Cholesterol: 0mg Sodium: 70mg Total Carbohydrates: 19g Dietary Fiber: 4g Sugars: 14g Protein: 4g

The benefits of this diet:

- Good source of antioxidants: Berries are a good source of antioxidants, which can help protect against cellular damage and support overall health.

- Supports healthy fats: The olive oil in the dressing is a good source of monounsaturated fats, which can help lower cholesterol levels and promote heart health.

- Supports weight management: The fiber in the spinach and berries can help support weight management by promoting feelings of fullness and reducing overall calorie intake.

- Supports blood sugar control: The honey in the dressing provides a natural source of sweetness, which can help support blood sugar control.

Broccoli Apple and Almond Salad Recipe

Preparation Time: 10 minutes

Servings: 2

Ingredients:

- 2 cups broccoli florets
- 1 medium apple, chopped
- 1/4 cup sliced almonds
- 2 tablespoons raisins
- 2 tablespoons lemon juice
- 2 tablespoons olive oil
- 1 teaspoon honey
- salt and pepper, to taste

Instructions:

1. In a large bowl, mix together the broccoli florets, chopped apple, sliced almonds, and raisins.

2. In a small bowl, whisk together the lemon juice, olive oil, honey, salt, and pepper until well combined.

3. Pour the dressing over the mixed greens mixture and toss until evenly coated.

4. Cover the bowl with plastic wrap and refrigerate for at least 30 minutes to allow the flavors to develop.

5. Serve the broccoli apple and almond salad chilled and enjoy!

Nutritional Information (per serving): Calories: 250 Total Fat: 18g Saturated Fat: 2g Cholesterol: 0mg Sodium: 75mg Total Carbohydrates: 21g Dietary Fiber: 5g Sugars: 14g Protein: 5g

The benefits of this diet:

- Good source of vitamins and minerals: Broccoli is a good source of vitamins C and K, and the apple provides a good source of vitamin C.

- Supports healthy fats: The olive oil in the dressing is a good source of monounsaturated fats, which can help lower cholesterol levels and promote heart health.

- Supports weight management: The fiber in the broccoli and apple can help support weight management by promoting feelings of fullness and reducing overall calorie intake.

- Supports blood sugar control: The honey in the dressing provides a natural source of sweetness, which can help support blood sugar control.

Ambrosia Salad Recipe

Preparation Time: 10 minutes

Servings: 2

Ingredients:

- 1 can (11 oz.) of mandarin oranges, drained
- 1 cup of chopped fresh pineapple
- 1 cup of small marshmallows
- 1/2 cup of shredded coconut
- 1/2 cup of plain nonfat Greek yogurt
- 1 tablespoon of honey
- 1 teaspoon of vanilla extract
- 1/4 cup of chopped pecans

Instructions:

1. In a large bowl, mix together the mandarin oranges, chopped pineapple, marshmallows, and shredded coconut.

2. In a small bowl, whisk together the Greek yogurt, honey, and vanilla extract.

3. Pour the yogurt mixture over the fruit mixture and stir until evenly coated.

4. Cover the bowl with plastic wrap and refrigerate for at least 30 minutes to allow the flavors to develop.

5. Before serving, sprinkle the chopped pecans on top of the ambrosia salad.

6. Serve chilled and enjoy!

Nutritional Information (per serving): Calories: 240 Total Fat: 9g Saturated Fat: 4g Cholesterol: 0mg Sodium: 80mg Total Carbohydrates: 40g Dietary Fiber: 2g Sugars: 32g Protein: 6g

The benefits of this diet:

- Good source of vitamins and minerals: Mandarin oranges and pineapple provide a good source of vitamin C, which is important for immune system support and skin health.

- Supports healthy fats: The pecans in the ambrosia salad provide a good source of monounsaturated and polyunsaturated fats, which can help lower cholesterol levels and promote heart health.

- Supports blood sugar control: The honey in the dressing provides a natural source of sweetness, which can help support blood sugar control.

- Supports digestive health: The fiber in the fruit mixture can help promote regularity and support digestive health.

Made in the USA
Monee, IL
09 November 2024